This essential handbook on in vitro fertilization provides an overview of gamete biology combined with a practical account and full description of the advanced technologies and protocols used in the modern fertility laboratory. The first section of the book describes how gametes are produced, their interaction and the first stages of embryo development. This foundation in gamete biology is essential background for the clinical embryologist wishing to implement a successful IVF programme. The laboratory protocols described in the second half of the book are clearly illustrated and cover the full range of techniques applied in IVF: semen analysis and preparation, oocyte retrieval and embryo culture, embryo freezing and thawing, and ICSI.

This is an indispensable and practical guide for clinical embryologists and indeed all clinical and laboratory staff involved in IVF.

In vitro fertilization

In vitro fertilization

BRIAN DALE
Director of Research, Stazione Zoologia, Naples

and

KAY ELDER
Director of Training, Bourn Hall Clinic, Cambridge

CAMBRIDGE UNIVERSITY PRESS

PUBLISHED BY THE PRESS SYNDICATE OF THE UNIVERSITY OF CAMBRIDGE
The Pitt Building, Trumpington Street, Cambridge CB2 1RP, United Kingdom

CAMBRIDGE UNIVERSITY PRESS
The Edinburgh Building, Cambridge, CB2 2RU, United Kingdom
40 West 20th Street, New York, NY 10011-4211, USA
10 Stamford Road, Oakleigh, Melbourne 3166, Australia

© Cambridge University Press 1997

This book is in copyright. Subject to statutory exception and to the provisions of relevant collective licensing agreements, no reproduction of any part may take place without the written permission of Cambridge University Press.

First published 1997
Reprinted 1998

Printed in the United Kingdom at the University Press, Cambridge

Typeset in 11/14 Monotype Times   [SE]

A catalogue record for this book is available from the British Library

Library of Congress Cataloguing in Publication data
Dale, Brian.
    In vitro fertilization / Brian Dale and Kay Elder.
        p.   cm.
    Includes bibliographical references.
    ISBN 0 521 57567 2 (pbk.)
    1. Fertilization in vitro, Human.   2. Fertilization in vitro.
    3. Germ Cells.   4. Fertilization (Biology)   I. Elder, Kay, 1946–
.   II. Title.
    [DNLM: 1. Fertilization in Vitro – methods.   2. Germ Cells – growth
    & development.   3. Fetal Development.   WQ 205D139i   1997]
    RG135.D34   1997
    618.1′78059–dc21
    DNLM/DLC 96–30056   CIP
    for Library of Congress

ISBN 0 521 57567 2 paperback

Every effort has been made in preparing this book to provide accurate and up-to-date information which is in accord with accepted standards and practice at the time of publication. Nevertheless, the authors, editors and publisher can make no warranties that the information herein is totally free from error, not least because clinical standards are constantly changing through research and regulation. The authors, editors and publisher therefore disclaim all liability for direct or consequential damages resulting from the use of the material contained in this book. The reader is strongly advised to pay careful attention to information provided by the manufacturer of any drugs or equipment that they plan to use.

Contents

	Preface	*page* xiii
1	Introduction	1
	Further reading	6
2	Producing gametes	8
	Oocyte growth	8
	Follicle cells	9
	Storage of informational molecules	9
	The regional organization of the oocyte	11
	Oocyte maturation	12
	Oogenesis in mammals	14
	Spermatogenesis in mammals	15
	Further reading	17
3	Sperm–oocyte interaction	19
	The acrosome and the vitelline coat	19
	Factors limiting sperm–oocyte fusion	21
	Activation of the spermatozoon	24
	Motility	24
	Chemotaxis	25
	Capacitation	25
	Acrosome reaction	27
	Activation of the oocyte and cell cycle regulation	27
	The cortical reaction and structural reorganization	31
	Events leading to the formation of the zygote nucleus	36
	The formation and fusion of the pronuclei	37
	Sperm–oocyte interaction in mammals	38
	Further reading	45

viii   *Contents*

4   First stages of development   46
    Cleavage patterns   46
    Cytoplasmic segregation and the formation of cell lines   48
    The segregation of somatic and germ cell lines in *Ascaris*   50
    First stages of development in mammals   50
    Further reading   52

5   Endocrine control of reproduction   55
    Further reading   56

6   Assisted reproductive technology (ART) in farm animals   58
    Further reading   66

7   Micromanipulation, assisted reproductive technology,
        and the future   67
    Further reading   72

8   The clinical in vitro fertilization laboratory   73
    Introduction   73
    Setting up a laboratory: equipment and facilities   74
    Tissue culture media   78
    Quality control procedures   79
    Tissue culture systems   80
    Basic equipment required for the IVF laboratory   82
    Further reading   83

9   Semen analysis and preparation for assisted
        reproductive techniques   85
    Semen assessment   85
    Preparation of sperm for in vitro fertilization/GIFT/ intrauterine
        insemination   89
    Sperm preparation for ICSI   97
    Retrograde ejaculation and electroejaculation: sperm
        preparation   99
    Sperm preparation: equipment and materials   99
    Further reading   100

10 Oocyte retrieval and embryo culture   102
    Programmed superovulation protocols   102
    Preparation for each case   105
    Oocyte retrieval (OCR) and identification   106
    Insemination   110
    Scoring of fertilization on day 1   111
    Embryo quality and selection for transfer   115

	Embryo transfer	120
	Gamete intrafallopian transfer (GIFT)	122
	Transport IVF	124
	Coculture systems	125
	Further reading	127
11	Cryopreservation	132
	Embryo freezing and thawing	132
	Blastocyst freezing	139
	Clinical aspects of frozen embryo transfer	141
	Oocyte cryopreservation	144
	Semen cryopreservation	144
	Further reading	147
12	Micromanipulation techniques	150
	Intracytoplasmic sperm injection	150
	Equipment for ICSI	160
	Adjustment of Narishige manipulators for ICSI	161
	Microtool preparation	168
	Assisted hatching	176
	Further reading	179
	Index	181

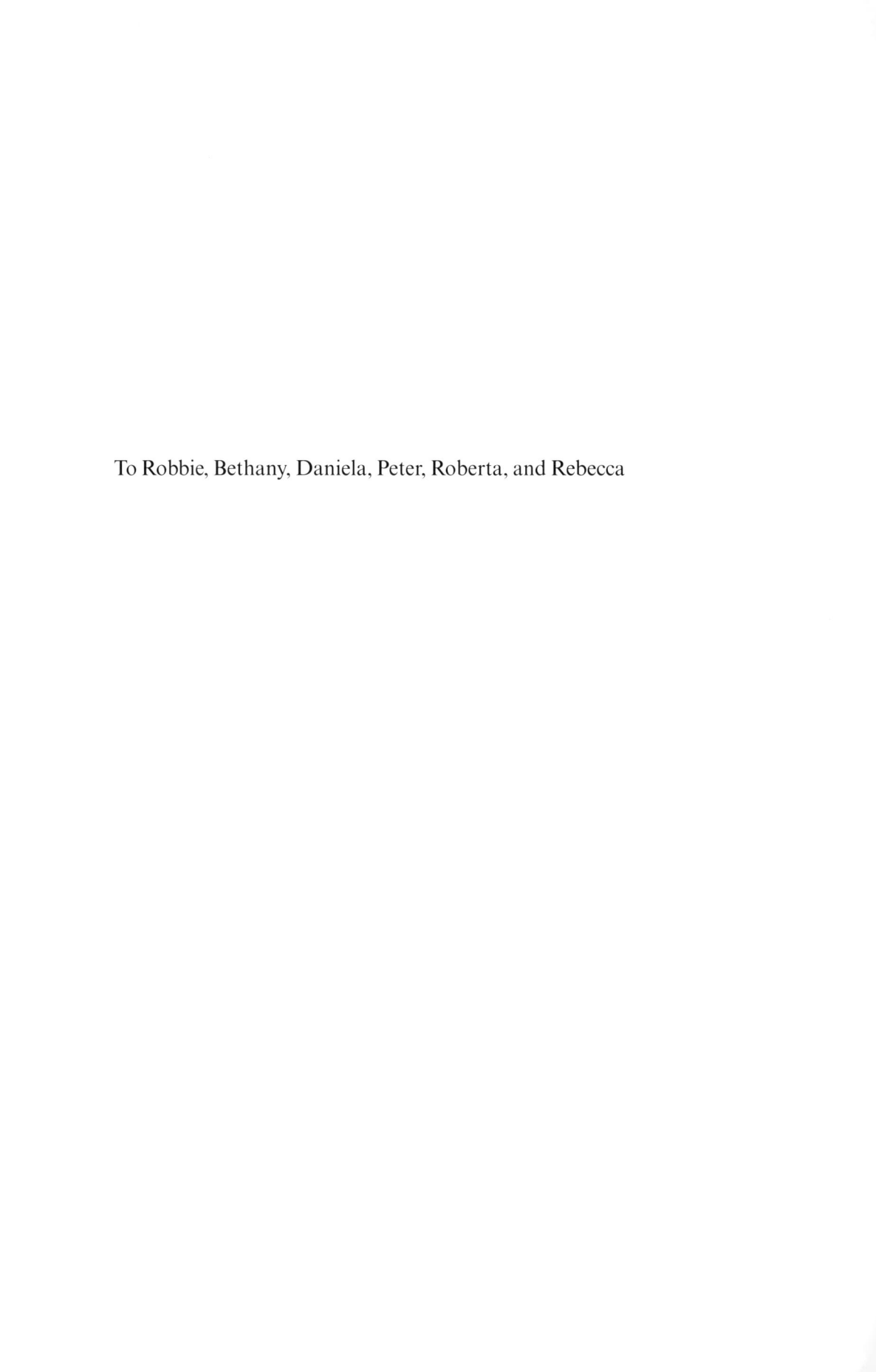

To Robbie, Bethany, Daniela, Peter, Roberta, and Rebecca

Preface

Since the birth of Louise Brown in 1978, there are now over 300 000 IVF children worldwide. Technology in assisted human reproduction is striding ahead; from the first births using frozen embryos in the early 1980s to sex-selection of embryos and the micro-injection of spermatozoa for the treatment of male sterility at the beginning of the present decade. However, research on human gametes and embryos, for various political and ethical reasons, has not followed suit. Although the clinical embryologist must be trained in standard cell culture technology, we believe it is equally important to be aware of the basic biology of these highly specialised cells, the gametes. Most of our information on gametes and early embryos has come from studies on invertebrates, less so from mammals, and therefore we have given a general overview of gamete biology, ending each chapter with a more specific description of mammalian and, where possible, human gamete biology.

The first part of this book explores how gametes are produced, how they interact, and the first steps of embryo development. The middle section is dedicated to the technologies used in animal ART and advanced laboratory technologies, whilst in the latter half of this book is a compilation of protocols used at Bourn Hall Clinic, Cambridge. The protocols were originally established in 1980 by Professor RG Edwards and Jean Purdy, following the years of research in the Cambridge University Department of Physiology and Kershaws Hospital in Oldham. Over the years they have been revised and adapted by many members of staff, all of whom are represented in the Further reading lists.

This book is one of the teaching elements used as part of the syllabus leading towards a Master of Science degree in Clinical Embryology at Anglia Polytechnic University, Cambridge, UK. The syllabus for this degree has been developed in conjunction with Alpha (Scientists in Reproductive Medicine).

B.D.
K.E.

1
Introduction

The last decade has seen a revival of interest in reproductive biology, owing in part to the successful application of gamete and embryo culture to medical, veterinary, and biotechnology practices, and in part to the pressing needs of today's society. In medical science, assisted reproductive technologies (ART) have been developed primarily to alleviate sterility, while in agricultural sciences the growing needs of the booming world population has provided the impetus to improve the efficiency of livestock production. The earliest documented use of ART was in 1783 when Spallazani delivered pups from an artificially inseminated bitch, but it was not until the 1900s that the Russian School of Ivanov developed artificial vaginas and insemination techniques to be used in horses, cattle, and sheep. The value of artificial insemination in farm animals depends upon the fact that the male ejaculate contains many millions of spermatozoa, theoretically sufficient to inseminate hundreds of females. A major leap forward in this direction was made in the late 1940s, when the team led by Chis Polge in Cambridge, England, developed techniques to freeze and store animal spermatozoa. This same period of time also saw the development of methods to isolate and manipulate the female gamete. In fact, in vitro maturation of mammalian oocytes was first reported by Pincus over 50 years ago, when it was observed that the primary oocyte of the rabbit resumed meiosis spontaneously when liberated from its follicle and placed in a suitable culture medium. It was not, however, until 1968 that Joe Sreenan in Ireland observed nuclear maturation in vitro in bovine oocytes recovered from slaughterhouse cattle. Although experiments on animals have traditionally preceded human studies, this has not always been the case in reproductive biology, where many of the new techniques and breakthroughs have been made using human gametes.

In nature, efficient reproduction relies on the synchronized behaviour of animals, the synchronized physiology of their reproductive organs and the synchronized interaction of the male and female gametes. This fundamental principle of synchronization has to be respected in ART, irrespective of the technique or species involved.

Fertilization marks the creation of a new and unique individual. It ensures immortality by transferring genetic information from one generation to the next and, by creating variation, allows evolutionary forces to operate. In addition to delivering the paternal genome, the spermatozoon triggers the quiescent female gamete into metabolic activity, essential to sustain early embryogenesis. Many texts portray fertilization as a process of activation and penetration of a large cell by a small cell. On the contrary, fertilization is a highly specialized example of cell–to–cell interaction, where each gamete activates its partner. Thus, to trigger metabolic activation of the oocyte, the spermatozoon itself must encounter and respond to signals originating from the oocyte and its investments. Sperm–oocyte interaction is a complex multistep process that starts with the specific recognition of complementary receptors on the surfaces of the two gametes and terminates with syngamy, the union of the maternal and paternal chromosomes. The central event is fusion of the plasma membranes of the two cells.

Both activation of the spermatozoon and activation of the oocyte are regulated by changes in intracellular messengers such as Ca^{2+}, H^+, cyclic adenosine monophosphate (cAMP), and inositol 1,4,5-trisphosphate (IP3). Intracellular Ca^{2+} may increase both by its release from intracellular stores and by flux through voltage-gated and chemical-gated channels in the plasma membrane.

Alberto Monroy in 1956 was one of the first to recognize the importance of ion fluxes through the plasma membrane in the process of oocyte activation, demonstrating a change in K^+ conductance in the starfish oocyte plasma membrane. In addition to the role of transmembrane voltage in the activation of both the oocyte and the spermatozoon, electrical recording from the former has made it possible to correlate the structural and physiological events of fertilization. There are two current hypotheses as to how a spermatozoon triggers the oocyte into metabolic activity:

1. A soluble factor in the spermatozoon may be released into the oocyte following gamete fusion.
2. Prior to fusion the interaction between the spermatozoon and a receptor on the oocyte surface is transduced to the oocyte interior via G-proteins or tyrosine kinase.

Although gametes from a particular batch from any individual animal appear to be homogeneous, they are in fact an extremely heterogeneous population of cells. Physiological parameters, ranging from the number of ion channels expressed in the plasma membrane, to the amount of Ca^{2+} released into the cytosol during activation, may vary 10-fold from cell to cell. With respect to viability, it has been estimated that in the sea urchin, for example, only 2% of spermatozoa are actually capable of fertilization. While in vitro techniques have made it possible for us to study the fertilization process in many animals, animal studies have also given rise to many misleading concepts. To date our knowledge of human gametes is scant and we therefore must look for guidance by resorting to information from animal models. This may be feasible at the physiological level, where we should seek to identify unifying concepts, but care must be taken when extrapolating data at the molecular level.

The first phase in the sexual reproduction of animals is called gametogenesis. This is a process of transformation whereby certain cells become the highly specialized sex cells: spermatogenesis in the male and oogenesis in the female. In both male and female, the primordial germ cells originate outside the gonad; once within the gonad they divide by mitosis to increase their number. This proliferation is followed by a period of cell growth which is much more significant in the female gamete than in the male gamete. The key event of gametogenesis, in both sexes, is the halving of the number of chromosomes during meiosis (Figure 1.1); thus in humans, where the chromosome number of somatic cells is 46, each oocyte and each spermatozoon has only 23 chromosomes; the similarity between oogenesis and spermatogenesis ends at this point. In the male, each primary spermatocyte divides meiotically to produce four spermatids, each of which becomes a functional spermatozoon, whereas in the female, of the four cells produced from each primary oocyte, only one develops into a viable oocyte (Figure 1.2). An unequal distribution of cytoplasm at division results in the production of three small cells, the polar bodies, which eventually degenerate.

A further distinction between the two gametes is that the spermatozoon acquires the ability to fertilize the oocyte only following the completion of meiosis; in the majority of animals, the oocyte is capable of interacting with the spermatozoon before meiosis is complete. In fact, meiosis in oocytes is arrested at various stages of the division cycle, depending upon the species, and is re-initiated as a result of fertilization (Figure 1.3). The sea urchin and some coelenterates are exceptions to this rule, in that their oocytes have completed meiosis before fertilization. Strictly speaking only in these two cases may the female gametes at the time of fertilization be termed ripe eggs; in all other cases they should be considered as oocytes. The process whereby the oocyte attains the ability to interact with spermatozoa, described by Delage in 1901 as cytoplasmic maturation, seems to be independent of the nuclear division cycle. It should be noted, however, that in oocytes which are normally fertilized before

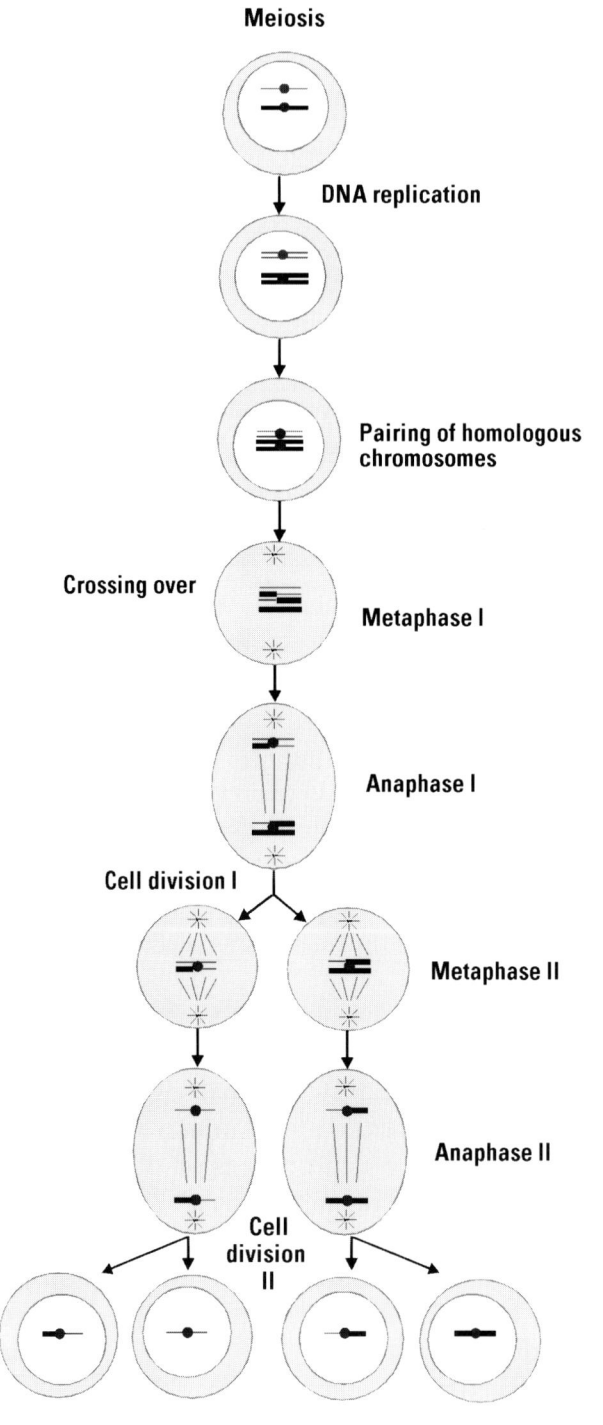

Figure 1.1 Meiosis. Four chromosomally unique haploid cells are generated from each diploid cell.

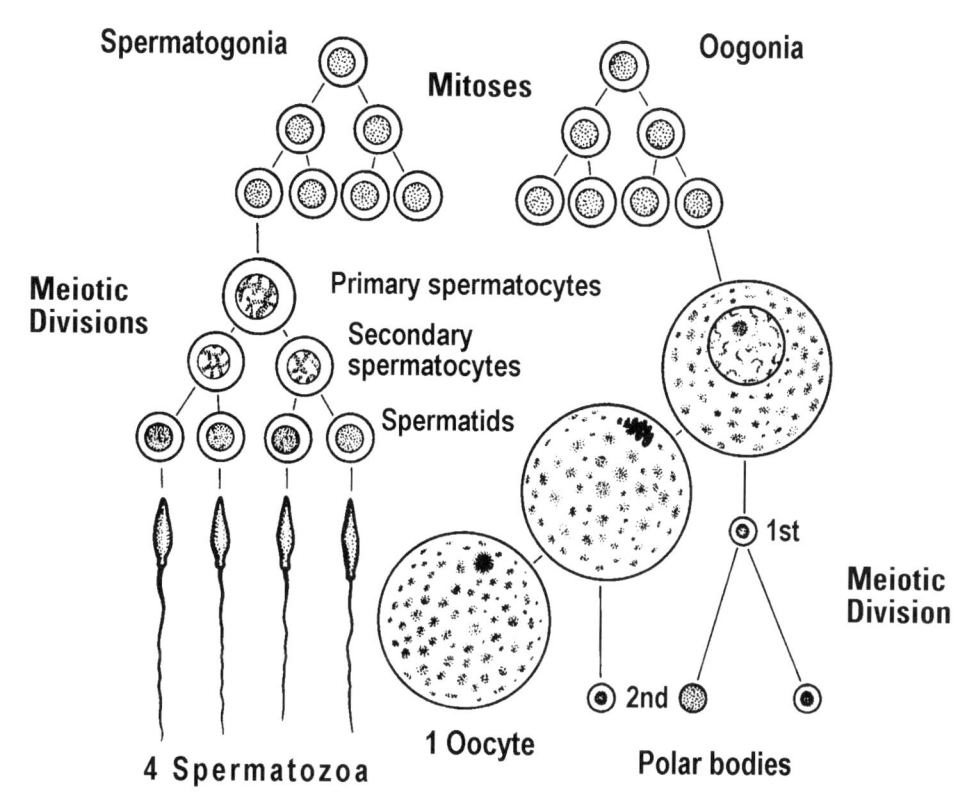

Figure 1.2 Gametogenesis in the male gives rise to four functional spermatozoa, while in the female only one of the four daughter cells becomes a functional oocyte. Modified from Dale (1983).

the completion of meiosis, the male nucleus remains quiescent in the cytoplasm until meiosis is completed.

The volume of a spermatozoon is a mere fraction of that of the oocyte; however, spermatozoa are often extremely long cells, reaching some 40 μm in sea urchins, 2–5 mm in some amphibia and 12 mm in some insects. There is great variation in the shape of spermatozoa, but, at the risk of over-simplifying, we may regard them morphologically and functionally to be composed of four regions : (1) the head containing the nucleus and the acrosome, (2) the neck containing the centrioles, (3) the middle piece, containing mitochondria, and (4) the tail piece or flagellum. Essentially the spermatozoon is a very compact cell with a few highly specialized cytoplasmic structures, including the flagellum for motility, and the acrosome which is instrumental in sperm–oocyte binding and fusion.

The size of oocytes also shows great variation: in marine invertebrates oocytes are about 60–150 μm in diameter, in mammals about 100 μm and in fish and

Prophase of 1st division	Metaphase of 1st division	Metaphase of 2nd division	Maturation complete
Nereis (Annellid)	*Chaetopterus* (Annellid)	Amphibians	Sea urchins
Pomatoceros (Annellid)	Ascidians	Fish	Coelenterates
Spisula (Mollusc)		Mammals	

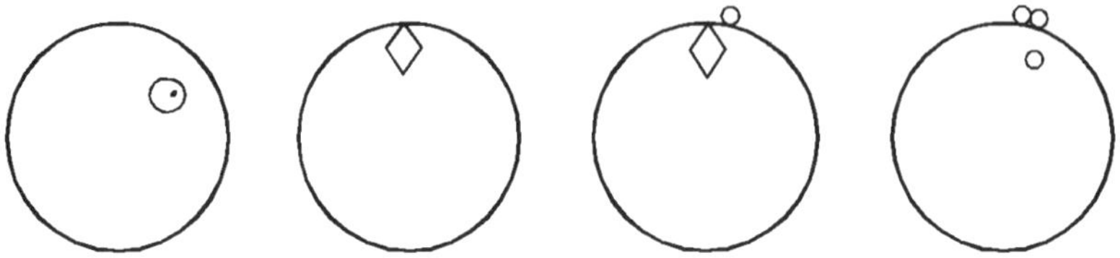

Figure 1.3 The different stages of meiotic arrest in oocytes from various species. Modified from Dale (1983).

amphibia about 1 mm. We are all familiar with the dimensions of bird eggs. Despite these differences in size, some generalities about their structure are apparent.

During the growth phase of oogenesis there is an intense synthesis of RNA and, to a lesser extent, of proteins; in other words the material to support early post-fertilization development of the embryo is formed. Typical cytoplasmic components of oocytes are yolk granules, pigment granules and mitochondria; cortical granules, a layer of membrane-bound vesicles located immediately beneath the plasma membrane, are common to many oocytes. Most oocytes are surrounded by several extracellular coats. The innermost layer is a fibrous glycoprotein sheet which plays a crucial role in sperm–oocyte interaction: this is known as the vitelline coat in echinoderms and amphibians, the chorion in ascidians and the zona pellucida in mammals. A variety of structures lie external to this: the jelly layer in sea urchins and amphibians, the follicle cells in ascidians and the cumulus oophorus (which also consists of follicle cells) in mammals. Finally, in birds and reptiles we find the tough, outer, inorganic shells, which are deposited around the oocyte after fertilization. All the extracellular components, apart from the inorganic shells, are present at fertilization, and therefore in order to fuse with the oocyte plasma membrane the spermatozoon has to interact with and traverse these outer layers.

Further reading

Austin, C.R. (1965) *Fertilization.* Prentice-Hall, New Jersey.
Austin, C.R. & Short, R.V. (1972) *Germ Cells and Fertilization.* Cambridge University Press, Cambridge.

Further reading

Balinsky, B.I. (1965) *An Introduction to Embryology*. Saunders, London.
Bodmer, C.W. (1968) *Modern Embryology*. Holt, Rinehart and Winston, New York.
Dale, B. (1983) *Fertilization in Animals.* Edward Arnold, London
Metz, C. & Monroy, A. (1985) *Biology of Fertilization*, Academic Press, New York.
Wassarman, P. (1987) The biology and chemistry of fertilization. *Science* **235**: pp. 553–560.

2
Producing gametes

Oocyte growth

The growth period of oocytes is usually quite long and the increase in size is often dramatic: the frog oocyte is an extreme example of this. The young oocyte, with a diameter of less than 50 µm, grows over a period of 3 years to reach a final diameter of 1500 µm. This represents an increase in size by a factor of over 20 000. Mammalian oocytes are much smaller, with a different time scale in their growth period, of weeks rather than years; however the increase in size is also considerable. For example, the mouse oocyte grows from some 20 µm to a final diameter of 70 µm, an increase in size by a factor of 40. It is fair to say that all oocytes are large and certainly larger than the average somatic cell which is usually about 10 µm in diameter. The size of the full grown oocyte depends principally on the amount of stored foodstuffs in the cytoplasm, although the nucleus also enlarges to some extent. The characteristic nucleus of the immature oocyte is called the germinal vesicle. Yolk is the major food storage product, although large quantities of lipid and glycogen granules are also found in some oocytes. The chemical composition of yolk varies from species to species according to its protein:fat ratio. In invertebrates and lower vertebrates yolk is usually found in the form of small granules, evenly distributed throughout the cytoplasm and contributing to around 20–30% of the total oocyte volume. Amphibian yolk, by contrast, contributes up to 80% of the oocyte volume and is organized into large flattened platelets. These platelets vary in size and are unequally distributed throughout the cytoplasm, the majority of the yolk lying at one pole: the vegetal pole. In teleost fish, birds and reptiles the yolk forms a compact central mass surrounded by a thin surface layer of cytoplasm with the nucleus in a thickened cytoplasmic cap at one end of the oocyte: the animal pole. Insect oocytes are similar but, in addition to the peripheral layer of cytoplasm, there is an internal mass of cytoplasm which contains the nucleus. In many animals the material stored in the oocyte during growth appears to be synthesized in parts of the body distinct from the ovary and carried to the ovary in soluble form via the blood stream. For example, in vertebrates yolk proteins and phospholipids are produced in the liver. Once inside the oocyte, these soluble yolk precursors are processed into insoluble yolk granules by the Golgi apparatus.

Follicle cells

During growth and maturation oocytes are surrounded by a layer, or layers, of specialized somatic cells called follicle cells. The oocyte and its follicle cells are in close association: studies with the electron microscope reveal the presence of gap junctions between the apposing membranes. These intercellular junctions, common also to many somatic tissues, serve as communicating devices through which ions and small molecules may pass. In the later stages of growth the oocyte develops numerous microvilli, presumably to maintain a functional surface area:volume ratio. A dense fibrillar material appears between the oocyte and its follicle cells, apparently secreted by the oocyte itself, which becomes the primary envelope: the vitelline coat. At this stage the follicle cells remain in contact with the oocyte by means of long microvilli interdigitating with the microvilli of the oocyte. At light microscopy, this microvillous zone has the appearance of a radially striated layer and has long been known in mammals as the zona radiata. In some animals, e.g. echinoderms and mammals, the microvilli are withdrawn to some extent shortly before ovulation, resulting in a continuous vitelline coat; in others, such as bivalve molluscs, the vitelline coat remains perforated by the microvilli. The follicle cells serve to transfer materials used in oocyte growth and also provide signals to trigger the oocyte into maturation.

Storage of informational molecules

In addition to foodstuffs, the oocyte accumulates specific informational macromolecules during growth which will serve later in the control of early embryogenesis. For example, considerable quantities of ribonucleic acids (RNAs) are present. In animal cells there are three main classes of RNA, designated messenger RNA (mRNA), transfer RNA (tRNA) and ribosomal RNA (rRNA); all three are involved in the synthesis of protein, and the relative amounts of the three types of RNA present vary from species to species. In the amphibian *Xenopus* there is a considerable synthesis of rRNA during oogenesis, which falls off during maturation and is then undetectable until the beginning of gastrulation. This means that the ribosomes in the oocyte are present in sufficient quantity to support protein synthesis in an embryo containing many thousand of cells. How does the oocyte manage to synthesize such a huge amount of rRNA, corresponding to the total synthesis of some 200 000 liver cells? In amphibians, this is achieved by a process called gene amplification: the rRNA genes are replicated many times over, forming several hundred copies. The germinal vesicle of the *Xenopus* oocyte contains many nucleoli; each nucleolus contains rRNA genes and is a site of rRNA synthesis. This mechanism of producing large amounts of rRNA in a relatively short period is by no means universally adopted, although gene amplification has also been detected in some invertebrate oocytes. In some insects, e.g. *Drosophila*, the nurse cells actively synthesize RNA which is then transferred to the oocyte by the cytoplasmic connections.

In the giant silk worm *Antheraea*, the DNA of the oocyte does not participate at all in RNA synthesis, and all of the RNA stored in the oocyte is synthesized by the nurse cells. This nurse cell–oocyte cooperation is certainly of great interest – but we should not forget that these two cell types are of common origin. Not all oocytes store large quantities of RNA. Mammalian oocytes contain a lesser amount of stored RNA, and new RNA is synthesized shortly after the second cleavage division. In the immature oocytes of some vertebrates and invertebrates the diplotene chromosomes are extremely elongated with thin loops extending from the main axis – these are known as lampbrush chromosomes. The loops of lampbrush chromosomes are known to be sites of intense RNA and protein synthesis, and the RNA:DNA ratio is over 100 times the RNA:DNA ratio found in liver chromatin. The base content of loop RNA is not comparable to that of rRNA, but resembles DNA, suggesting that it is in fact messenger RNA. What is the significance of this large quantity of mRNA? First, it appears that the vast majority of mRNA is retained in the embryo until the blastula stage to direct protein synthesis later in development. The mechanism by which it is made non-translatable until this late stage remains unknown, but it may be due to its association with proteins. Thus the oocyte at this stage contains a large amount of information which appears to be masked, but the rest of the protein synthesizing machinery is functional. This problem was approached by injecting foreign mRNA into oocytes. When rabbit haemoglobin mRNA was injected into amphibian oocytes, the oocytes synthesized rabbit haemoglobin; the more rabbit mRNA injected, the more haemoglobin was produced. The conclusion from this experiment is that the oocyte has the capacity to synthesize much more protein than it actually carries out, and that the amount of translatable mRNA is the limiting factor in protein synthesis. In addition, many proteins are synthesized during oogenesis but are set aside in the oocyte cytoplasm for use later on in development. For example, the enzymes necessary for DNA synthesis are present in the growing oocyte and yet DNA replication is switched off. Again the mechanism which inactivates these stored molecules remains a mystery.

The regional organization of the oocyte

The growing oocyte does not have an homogeneous structure; in particular, many cytoplasmic organelles become segregated to various regions of the oocyte and this regional organization determines some of the basic properties of the embryo. In all animal oocytes the pole where the nuclear divisions occur, resulting in the formation of the polar bodies, is called the animal pole. The opposite pole, which often contains a high concentration of nutrient reserves, is called the vegetal pole. Many cytoplasmic inclusions and organelles are distributed according to this animal–vegetal (A–V) axis: yolk is usually more dense at the vegetal pole than at the animal pole, and in some animals, particularly amphibians, there is a density gradient of pigment granules. The familiar unpigmented region of the frog oocyte is in fact the vegetal hemisphere. In cases where the heterogeneous organization of the cytoplasm cannot be detected, either by light or electron microscopy, it can usually be inferred from developmental studies. Some 50 years ago the Swedish zoologist S. Horstadius carried out classical experiments on the sea urchin oocyte, in which one species of Mediterranean sea urchin, *Paracentrotus lividus*, was found to have a band of red pigment just below the equator towards the vegetal pole. This was the marker used to orientate the oocyte. When this oocyte was cut with a fine glass needle along the animal–vegetal axis (which is the plane of the first cleavage division) the two halves rounded up forming two small cells. Both halves could be fertilized, and potentially gave rise to two normal plutei larvae. When the cut was equatorial, however, dividing the oocyte into animal and vegetal halves which were then fertilized, only the vegetal half gave rise to a complete pluteus. The animal half gave rise to a ciliated blastula-like sphere which was incapable of gastrulation.

The conclusion from these experiments was that in the unfertilized sea urchin oocyte there is an uneven distribution of factors along the A–V axis, which are essential for normal development. What are these factors: are they related to the regional organization of large cytoplasmic organelles, or are they freely diffusible molecules organized along an A–V gradient? Centrifugation of unfertilized oocytes yielded further information: the cytoplasmic components can be shifted by centrifugation at 3000 g to form layers according to their relative densities. From the centripetal pole a lipid layer, a layer of clear cytoplasm containing the nucleus, a layer of mitochondria, then yolk and finally pigment granules are found. The plane of the cytoplasmic stratification is randomly orientated with respect to the A–V axis and yet such centrifuged oocytes always develop into normal plutei. More convincingly, by increasing the centrifugal force to $10\,000\,g$ the oocytes actually break, first into halves, then quarters. Each quarter may be fertilized and will develop into a perfect larva. It seems likely therefore that those cytoplasmic organelles which may be displaced by centrifugation do not determine the A–V polarity of the oocyte. What are the alternatives? One possibility is that the oocyte cortex, including the plasma membrane, may be the determining factor. Generally speaking the cortex is rigid and granules within it, such as the cortical granules, cannot be displaced by centrifugation. This would explain the normal development of oocytes following the dramatic displacement of cytoplasmic organelles. All oocytes have a polarized organization and the embryo maintains this A–V axis throughout development; however, the axis is not always rigidly determined as in the sea urchin. For example, the unfertilized ascidian oocyte may be cut into two halves along any plane and yet both halves when fertilized will give rise to normal larvae. This indicates that the fragments are capable of reorganizing themselves and developing a new A–V axis. How does polarity originate? Unfortunately little information is available. In the molluscs *Dentalium* and *Lymnaea*, the process seems to be epigenetic; the area of contact between the oocyte and the ovary wall becomes the vegetal pole.

Finally, in addition to A-V polarity many oocytes express a bilateral symmetry either before fertilization, as in insects, or shortly afterwards, as in ascidian oocytes.

Oocyte maturation

Maturation is the third and final phase of oogenesis, during which several changes occur in the oocyte, preparing it for ovulation and its imminent interaction with a spermatozoon. Maturation involves nuclear, meiotic, and cytoplasmic events, including changes in the organization of the plasma membrane as a part of cytoplasmic maturation. Throughout the growth period the large oocyte nucleus (or germinal vesicle) is blocked in prophase of the first meiotic division. Breakdown of the nuclear membrane, resulting in the mixture of nucleoplasm and cytoplasm, is the first indication of maturation. The semi-contracted chromosomes, now in the cytoplasm, migrate to the periphery of the oocyte where they become arranged on the spindle. In most animals the meiotic cycle does not proceed to completion; the process is arrested a second time, usually at metaphase of the first or second division (see Fig. 1.3).

The oocyte is now ready to be ovulated, i.e. to be expelled from the ovary.

Shortly after ovulation, fertilization occurs and the interaction of the spermatozoon stimulates the resumption of meiosis. We may say therefore that in the majority of animals the processes of oocyte maturation and fertilization overlap. There are of course exceptions: the echinoids (sea urchins) and the coelenterates (anemones) lie at one extreme, where fertilization occurs after the oocyte has completed meiosis. At the other extreme are some marine worms where the process of oocyte maturation is in fact triggered by the fertilizing spermatozoon. In all oocytes which are normally fertilized before the completion of meiosis the sperm nucleus remains inactive in the cytoplasm until the oocyte ejects both polar bodies.

Oocyte maturation has been extensively studied in amphibians and starfish. Despite the diversity of these animals, the processes are remarkably similar and depend upon the production of hormones at sites distant from the ovary. In amphibians, gonadotrophic hormones secreted by the pituitary glands control maturation and ovulation, whereas in starfish the prime effector is a gonad-stimulating substance produced by the nervous system. Both hormones seem to have dual targets: they act initially on ovarian tissue inducing ovulation, and they subsequently stimulate follicle cells causing them to release a second factor or messenger which acts directly on the oocyte plasma membrane to induce the cellular process of maturation. In starfish this second messenger has been isolated and identified as 1-methyl-adenine. In amphibians it appears to be a progesterone-like molecule. A complex sequence of cytoplasmic events are set in motion following interaction of the secondary messenger with the oocyte plasma membrane and these lead to the breakdown of the germinal vesicle. Mammalian ovulation and maturation is also under the control of pituitary hormones, in particular follicle stimulating hormone (FSH) and luteinizing hormone (LH); however, the situation here is more complicated and requires the additional interplay of the ovarian hormones oestrogen and progesterone.

In the 1940s Lindahl and Holter demonstrated that the rate of oxygen consumption in sea urchin oocytes drops concurrently with the onset of maturation. This led to the general idea that oocyte metabolism is depressed during maturation and becomes reactivated as a result of fertilization. This seems to be the case in many animals, for example fish, ascidians, some worms and molluscs.

In contrast, in mammals, amphibians and starfish, maturation is a period of synthetic and metabolic activity. For example, hormone-induced maturation in starfish and amphibian oocytes leads to a five to tenfold increase in the rate of protein synthesis, and in amphibians and mammals the RNA synthesis which started so intensely during the growth phase continues throughout maturation. Not all of the metabolic processes are activated by the hormones. In the starfish, although protein synthesis is stimulated during maturation, oxygen consumption does not increase until fertilization. Although it is difficult to draw general conclusions, it appears that in cases of hormonally-induced maturation (for example amphibians and starfish) a part of the metabolic de-repression of the oocyte is induced by the hormones, and the remainder by the action of the fertilizing spermatozoon. In contrast, in all other cases (for example most invertebrates and fish) metabolic de-repression comes about solely as the result of fertilization.

Although controversy continues at the moment, it is generally thought that an increase in intracellular calcium is the trigger for re-initiation of meiosis. Maturation promoting factor (MPF) which consists of Cdc2 kinase and cyclin, and the Mos protein kinase (an essential component of cytostatic factor) are probably low in prophase 1 arrested oocytes and increase during oocyte maturation to reach a peak at the stage of metaphase arrest.

Oogenesis in mammals

The mitotic phase of germ cell proliferation in the human female terminates before birth, and by the fifth month of foetal life all oogonia have entered their first meiotic divison to become primary oocytes. At puberty a total of about 200 000 germ cells are available for her reproductive life-span. During the first meiotic prophase the oocytes are surrounded by mesenchymal ovarian cells to become primordial follicles. The oocytes arrest in diplotene with the characteristic large nucleus called the germinal vesicle. It is not known how these arrested oocytes remain viable for up to 50 years. Recruitment of some of these primordial follicles begins at puberty, when the recruited follicle grows from 20 μm to several hundred microns, and the oocyte itself grows from 10 μm to about 100 μm. The growth phase essentially involves synthesis and storage of large amounts of RNA, proteins and metabolic substrates. During this growth period, the surrounding granulosa cells divide mitotically, and the zona pellucida, a glycoprotein coat synthesised by the oocyte, is secreted between the oocyte and the cells. Gap junctions allow transfer of substrates and developmental information between the oocyte and the cytoplasmic projections of the accessory cells that penetrate the zona pellucida. The small number of follicles that have completed their growth phase are called pre-antral follicles, and many of these will undergo atresia. Circulating gonadotrophins convert the pre-antral follicles to antral follicles or Graffian follicles. The pre-antral phase lasts for 8–12 days in women, and during this phase fluid accumulates in the follicle which suspends the oocyte with surrounding cumulus cells. During this phase of growth the follicle produces an increased amount of androgens and oestrogens.

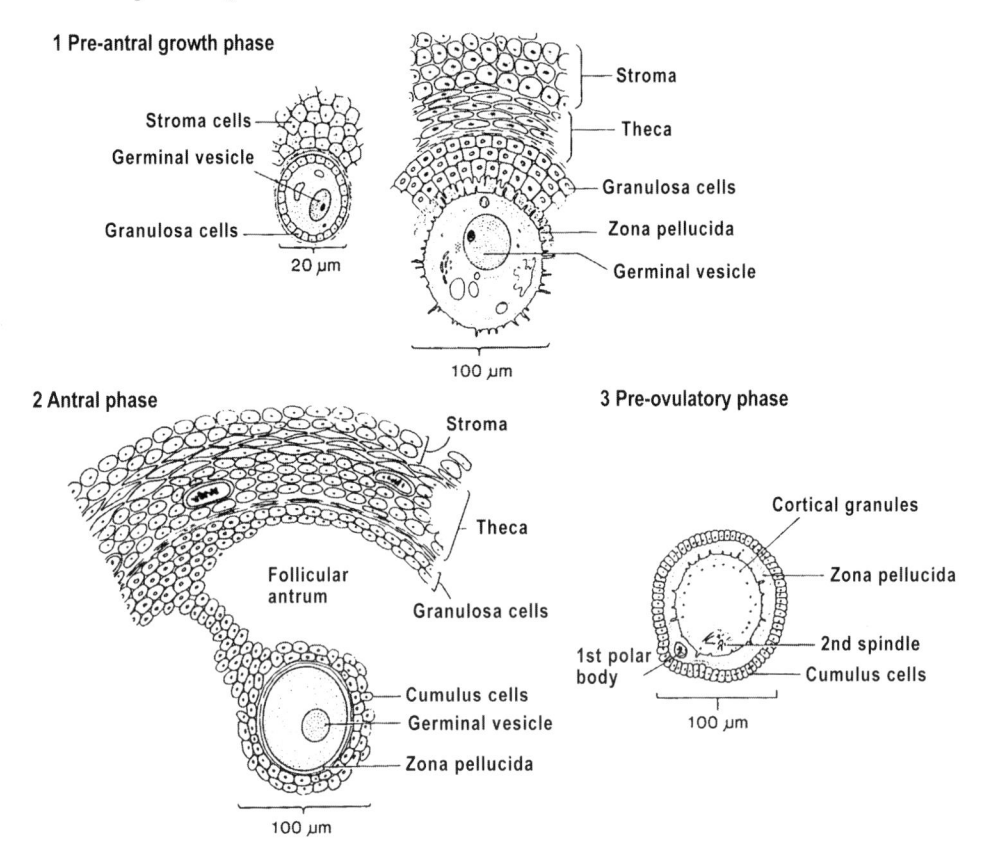

Figure 2.1 Oogenesis in the human. Modified from Johnson & Everitt (1990).

A subsequent surge of LH causes a rapid further accumulation of fluid, now called the pre-ovulatory phase of approximately 36 hours duration, leading to a 25 mm diameter follicle (in the human) which then ovulates. Fimbria of the oviduct are thought to sweep the ovulated oocyte into the oviductal ampulla where fertilization will occur. In this final maturation stage of oogenesis the nuclear membrane breaks down, meiosis is re-initiated and the first polar body is extruded. The female cell is now in the stage of second metaphase. Concomitantly, a process of cytoplasmic maturation is initiated, which includes a decrease in potassium conductance, a depolarization of the plasma membrane and migration of cortical granules to the surface of the oocyte (Figure 2.1).

Spermatogenesis in mammals

In the male, the interphase germ cells start to proliferate by mitoses at puberty. This is followed by meiosis and a gradual reorganization of cellular components, characterized by a loss of cytoplasm. In the adult mammal it has been estimated that about 500 spermatozoa per second are produced per gram of testis. The stem cells, or A0 spermatogonia, are located in the basal intratubular compartment. At intervals A-l spermatogonia emerge from this population and undergo a fixed number of mitotic divisions to form a clone of daughter cells. There is some evidence that one of the daughter clones serves as a second source of stem cells. After the final mitotic division the primary spermatocytes move into the adluminal compartment and enter into meiosis. In this compartment they undergo two meiotic divisions to form, first two daughter secondary spermatocytes, and eventually four early spermatids. Although spermatid nuclei contain haploid sets of chromosomes the autosomes continue to synthesize low levels of ribosomal and messenger RNA and proteins. The spermatid DNA now becomes highly condensed and is eventually packed with protamines. Cytoplasmic reorganization gives rise to the tail, the midpiece containing the mitochondria, the acrosome and the residual body which casts off excess cytoplasm. Sperm modelling is probably regulated by the Sertoli cells. As spermatogenesis proceeds, the cells are moved to the centre of the tubular lumen. In humans spermatogenesis is complete in 64 days. The rate of progression of cells through spermatogenesis is constant and unaffected by external factors such as hormones (Figure 2.2).

Mammalian spermatozoa leaving the testis are not capable of fertilizing oocytes. They gain this ability while passing down the epididymis, a process known as epididymal maturation. Testicular spermatozoa are essentially motionless, even when washed and placed in a physiological solution. The ability to move is probably regulated at the level of the plasma membrane, as de-membranation and exposure to ATP, cAMP and Mg^{2+} triggers movement. Transfer of a forward motility protein and carnitin from the epididymal fluid are believed to be important for the development of sperm motility. The osmolality and chemical composition of the epididymal fluid varies from one segment to the next, and it may be that the sperm plasma membrane is altered stepwise as it progresses down the duct. Then the spermatozoal head acquires the ability to adhere to the zona pellucida, with an increase in net negative charge. During maturation the spermatozoa use up endogenous reserves of metabolic substrates, becoming dependent on exogenous sources such as fructose, and they then shed their cytoplasmic droplet. When the sperm leaves the testis it is coated with several macromolecules which are either lost, altered or added to during passage through the epididymus. The most prominent molecules are glycoproteins mediated by galacto-transferase and sial-transferase. Changes in the lectin-binding ability of the sperm plasma membrane during

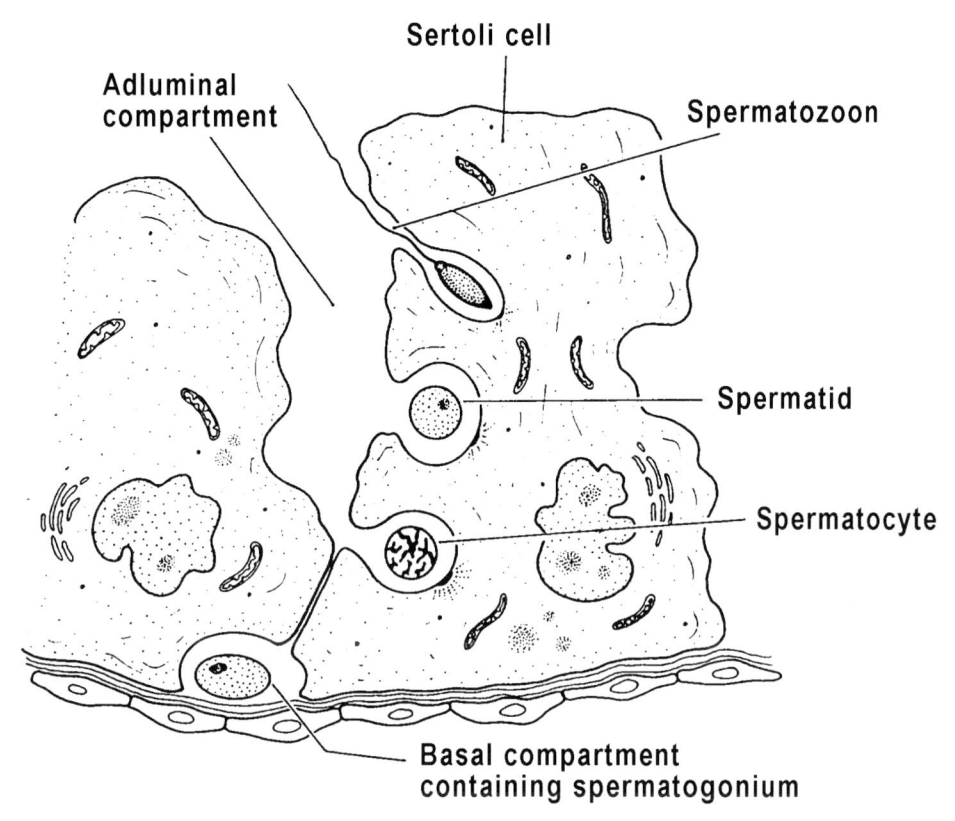

Figure 2.2 Spermatogenesis in the mammal. Maturation and modeling of the male gamete is regulated by the Sertoli cell. Modified after Johnson & Everitt (1990).

epididymal maturation indicate alterations to the terminal saccharide residues of these glycoproteins. Membrane lipids also undergo changes in their physical and chemical composition.

Further reading
Bellvé, A. & O'Brien, D (1983) In *Mechanism and Control of Animal Fertilization*. Academic Press, New York.
Dale, B. (1996) In: (Greger, R. Windhorst, U. eds), *Comprehensive Human Physiology*. Springer Verlag, Berlin.
Gurdon, J.B. (1967) On the origin and persistence of a cytoplasmic state inducing nuclear DNA synthesis in frog's eggs. *Proceedings of the National Academy of Science of the USA* **58**: 545–552.
Johnson, M. & Everitt, B. (1990) *Essential Reproduction*. Blackwell Scientific Publications, Oxford.
Masui, Y. (1985) In: (Metz, C.B. Monroy, A. eds), *Biology of Fertilization*. Academic Press, New York, pp. 189–219.

Nurse, P. (1990) Universal control mechanisms resulting the onset of M-phase. *Nature* **344**: 503–508.

Sagata, N. (1996)Meiotic metaphase arrest in animal oocytes: its mechanisms and biological significance *Trends in Cell Biology* **6**: 22–28.

Van Blerkom, J. & Motta, P. (1979) *The Cellular basis of Mammalian Reproduction*. Urban and Scwarzenberg.

Yanagimachi, R. (1994) Mammalian Fertilization. In: Knobil, E. & Neill, J. eds), *The Physiology of Reproduction*. Raven Press, New York, pp. 189–317.

3
Sperm–oocyte interaction

The acrosome and the vitelline coat

Fertilization is a complex process of cell–cell interaction which starts with the specific recognition and binding of spermatozoa to oocytes and ultimately leads to the fusion of the male and female pronuclei. The initial stages of fertilization depend principally on two structures: the acrosome of the spermatozoon (Figure 3.1) and the vitelline coat of the oocyte. For convenience, we may consider three major events in sperm–oocyte interaction:

1. Attachment of the spermatozoon to the vitelline coat.
2. The spermatozoon undergoes the acrosome reaction, as a result of which digestive enzymes are released and the inner acrosomal membrane is exposed.
3. This highly fusogenic sperm membrane makes contact with the oocyte plasma membrane and the two membranes fuse together.

The vitelline coat is composed of protein and carbohydrates in the form of glycoprotein units which are probably stabilized by disulphide bonds. Unfortunately, there is little biochemical information on this oocyte envelope; the principal carbohydrate appears to be fucose and the glycoprotein units are synthesized by the oocyte itself. The form of the vitelline coat varies greatly from species to species. For example, in the sea urchin the vitelline coat is very thin and adheres tightly to the oocyte surface following the contours of the surface microvilli, whereas in the starfish it is much thicker and is perforated by the microvilli. The situation in mammals and ascidians is quite different: the vitelline coat is extremely thick and in fact it may be removed manually using fine steel needles. In the ascidians the vitelline coat is actually separated from the oocyte surface by a layer of cells called test cells.

How does the spermatozoon attach to the vitelline coat and what is the molecular basis for this interaction? There are complementary molecules on the surface of the spermatozoal head and on the vitelline coat. Plant lectins such as concanavalin A and fucose binding protein, which are proteins that bind specifically to certain carbohydrates, bind both to the surface of the chorion and to the head of the spermatozoon in ascidians. Fucose is an important molecule in the process of gamete binding, as evidenced by the fact that the addition of this sugar to a mixture of spermatozoa and oocytes inhibits fertilization, i.e. fucose competitively inhibits sperm–oocyte interaction. Whatever the nature of the complementary structures, binding of the spermatozoon to the vitelline coat induces the acrosome reaction.

Turning now to the spermatozoon, consider the structure of the apically situated acrosome. Although again there is considerable variation between species, the acrosome of *Saccoglossus*, a hemichordate, is considered to be relatively typical. The membrane bound acrosomal granule, which contains lytic agents such as proteases, sulphatases and glycosidases is bound within the plasma membrane of the spermatozoon. When the spermatozoon attaches to the vitelline coat the permeability of the sperm plasma membrane is altered causing a transient change in the concentration of several intracellular ions, as a result of which the acrosome reaction is triggered. Using *Saccoglossus* as an example, four stages in the reaction may be considered:

1. The acrosome membrane fuses with the sperm plasma membrane at the tip of the acrosome.
2. The acrosomal granule breaks down releasing lysins. These enzymes either 'dissolve' a pathway through the vitelline coat or alter it in such a way as to allow the penetration of the acrosomal tubule.
3. This tubule is formed by the extension of the inner acrosomal membrane, by polymerization of actin or actin-like fibres located in the sub-acrosomal region.
4. When the tip of the acrosomal tubule contacts the oocyte plasma membrane the two membranes fuse.

In some animals an insoluble protein component of the acrosomal granule known as 'bindin' remains attached to the extended tubule during growth and is thought to be involved in the 'adhesion' of gametes. It is technically difficult to study the time sequence of these events, but the first two are thought to occur within 1 second while completion of the reaction (i.e. up to fusion of the two gametes) may take 7–9 seconds (for example in the annelid *Hydroides* and the hemichordate *Saccoglossus*).

Cytological investigations have revealed that the acrosome is of Golgi origin. The Golgi body in an early spermatid consists of a series of concentrically arranged membranes around an aggregation of small vesicles. One of the vesicles increases in size and fills with particulate material. Vesicle growth may come about as the result of fusion of several smaller vesicles. When the vesicle containing the future acrosomal granule reaches a certain size it migrates towards the nucleus. Shortly afterwards, the nucleus starts to elongate, the vesicle loses much of its fluid content and the vesicle membrane wraps around the front of the nucleus forming the typical acrosome. This generalized picture of sperm–oocyte interaction where the spermatozoon attaches to the vitelline coat with its acrosome intact and an acrosomal tubule is produced as part of the process is not universal. In starfish and sea cucumbers the acrosome reaction occurs when the spermatozoon contacts the outer surface of the jelly layer. Here the acrosomal tubule is extremely long, reaching 20 μm in the starfish and extends across the width of the jelly layer to make contact with the oocyte surface. In sea urchins, where the acrosome reaction occurs upon contact with the vitelline coat, the acrosomal tubule is very short, usually less than 1μm – not surprising, considering the close apposition of the vitelline coat and the plasma membrane in these oocytes. In mammals and ascidians the vitelline coat is very thick and, in the latter case, distant from the oocyte surface. Here the acrosome reaction also occurs upon contact of the spermatozoon with the vitelline coat, but an acrosomal tubule is not formed as part of the process. Finally, in bony fish, where the oocyte is covered by a thick chorion and the spermatozoon makes contact with the oocyte surface by way of a micropyle, the spermatozoon lacks an acrosome.

Factors limiting sperm–oocyte fusion

Although the oocyte is an extremely large cell it is by no means freely accessible to the spermatozoon. The extracellular coats and in some cases the heterogeneous organization of the oocyte itself limit the number of spermatozoa which are able to reach the oocyte surface. Before interacting with the vitelline coat the spermatozoa must traverse and interact with the outer oocyte investments, which in sea urchins, ascidians and mammals are the jelly layer, the follicle cells and the cumulus cells, respectively (Figure 3.2). All of these layers drastically reduce the number of spermatozoa which reach the underlying vitelline coat. In the sea urchin the jelly layer itself, particularly shortly after spawning when it is tough and compact, apparently induces a premature acrosome reaction and thereby reduces the number of viable sperm which reach the vitelline coat by up to 90%. In ascidians, spermatozoa can only react with restricted areas of the vitelline coat which are not covered by the follicle cells. Having traversed the outer investments, the spermatozoa must bind to and then penetrate the vitelline coat. It appears that not all of the bound sperm are able to do this, and many are not triggered into an acrosome reaction. This may be due to the heterogeneity of the glycoproteins in the vitelline coat. It is well

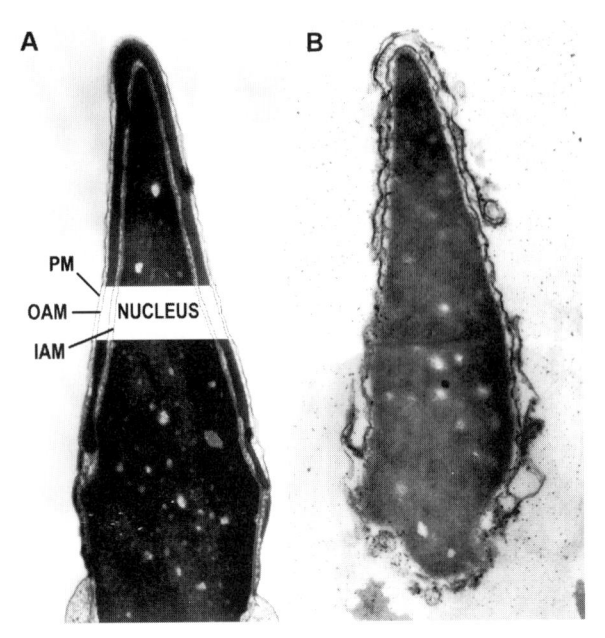

Figure 3.1 Transmission electron microscope (TEM) section through a human spermatozoon showing the plama membrane (pm) and outer (oam) and inner (iam) acrosomal membranes. To the right is a TEM of a human spermatozoon after exposure to the calcium ionophore A23187 has triggered the acrosome reaction.

accepted that the integral glycoproteins of cell membranes display a certain degree of microheterogeneity due to differential glycosylation, i.e. the sugar side chains of these molecules vary slightly. In order for sperm to attach to the vitelline coat, a specific molecular fit may be required to induce the acrosome reaction.

An additional factor limiting sperm–oocyte fusion is the organization of the oocyte plasma membrane. In some oocytes, sperm fusion is restricted to a limited area of the oocyte surface. In ascidians this occurs in a region of about 30 degrees at the vegetal pole, and can be demonstrated in live oocytes deprived of their vitelline coat. In amphibians the site of spermatozoal entry is restricted to the animal hemisphere. The most striking case is that of *Discoglossus* in which the site of interaction is limited to a small dimple at the animal pole. The fine structural organization of these sites is different from that of the rest of the egg surface. In *Xenopus* and *Rana* spermatozoa can be 'forced' to penetrate the vegetal pole, although such sperm are unable to develop into pronuclei. The restriction in area available for sperm penetration is of course most obvious in the case of oocytes with micropyles (i.e. fish, insects, squid). The diameter of the micropyle is usually the same as the head of the spermatozoon and as

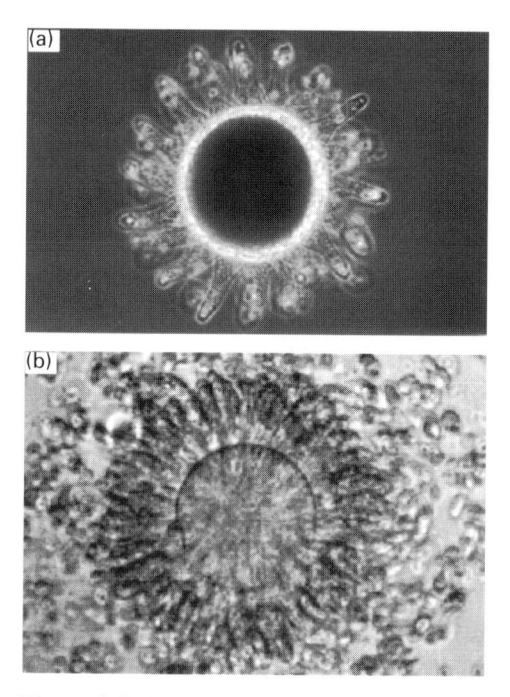

Figure 3.2 (a) Metaphase I oocyte of the ascidian *Ciona intestinalis* with its surrounding chorion and star-shaped follicle cells. (b) Metaphase II human oocyte with its corona–cumulus complex.

mentioned previously the spermatozoa lack an acrosome. In trout and other salmonids, when a spermatozoon reaches the oocyte plasma membrane the cortical alveoli begin to open and their contents form a plug in the micropyle. Thus only one spermatozoon is allowed to reach the oocyte surface.

In the course of evolution it appears that no method has been devised which allows the union of one spermatozoon with one oocyte without great wastage of spermatozoa. In most animals spermatozoa are produced in huge excess, irrespective of whether fertilization occurs externally in the sea or internally in the female tract. In humans the sperm–oocyte ratio can be as high as 10^9:1 and in the sea urchin 10^4:1. Despite these high ratios, behavioural adaptations are also necessary to ensure fertilization: in the case of echinoderms and some polychaetes, this takes the form of aggregation of mature animals and the simultaneous spawning of the sexes. In aquatic animals dilution of gametes in the surrounding medium and loss to predators greatly reduces the probability of fertilization. In mammals, of the millions of spermatozoa ejaculated only a few reach the site of fertilization, which in most species is the ampullae of the fallopian tube. In a study of fertilization in the mouse in vivo a 1:1

sperm–oocyte ratio was discovered in the ampullae; supernumerary spermatozoa were never observed.

In other animals, notably insects and nematodes sperm utilization is much more efficient. In *Drosophila* there is a 1:1 relationship between the progeny recovered and the number of spermatozoa counted in the seminal receptacles. In hermaphrodite fertilization of the nematode *Caenorhabditis elegans* every spermatozoon fertilizes an oocyte; however, in this case not all oocytes are fertilized because the oocytes are produced in excess. The high efficiency of sperm utilization in insects and nematodes with internal fertilization may be an important adaptation as it enables volume to be minimized, and allows provision of nutrients for the stored spermatozoa. It seems therefore that in most animals, although great quantities of spermatozoa are produced very few reach the oocyte. Those that do then encounter the problem of penetrating the extracellular coats and fusing with the oocyte plasma membrane. Polyspermy, a lethal condition where several spermatozoa enter the oocyte, is probably rare in nature.

Activation of the spermatozoon

The majority of reports on sperm–oocyte interaction emphasize the activation of the oocyte by the spermatozoon; however, prior activation of the spermatozoon is a prerequisite for successful fertilization. Activation of the male gamete involves several behavioural, physiological and structural changes, some of which are induced at shedding by exposure to environmental signals, and others are induced whilst the spermatozoon is interacting with the oocyte and its extracellular investments. All of these changes are essential for successful fertilization.

Motility

Spermatozoa are maintained in the testis in a quiescent state. Many factors may be responsible for this metabolic suppression, such as physical restraint, low pH and low oxygen tension of the seminal fluid. In most marine invertebrates shedding of the spermatozoa into the sea induces motility, presumably by the reversal of the restraining conditions of the testes. Once released they are fervently active, and if they do not encounter an oocyte they rapidly deplete their energy supply and die. Their lifespan depends on their activity; generally speaking the less active they are the longer they live. In teleost fish, motility is also induced when the spermatozoa are shed into the aquatic environment; the triggering factor here is the tonicity of the new environment. In fresh-water fish, the external medium is hypotonic with respect to the seminal plasma whereas in marine fish it is hypertonic; therefore in the former species a hypotonic shock induces motility, and in the latter species a hypertonic shock is responsible. In salmonid fish the seminal plasma has a high K^+ content of about 80 mM which suppresses motility; when spermatozoa are shed the K^+ is diluted and sperm start to move about vigorously.

Chemotaxis

Once motile, the spermatozoon must encounter an oocyte before its energy reserves are depleted. Many mechanisms have evolved to facilitate gamete encounter, including the synchronization of gamete production and release, copulatory devices, and the production of chemical attractants by the ovary or oocytes. The phenomenon of chemotaxis in fertilization (the oriented movement of spermatoza in a chemical gradient), although an intuitively attractive mechanism, has only been demonstrated in a few animals, for example cnidarians and tunicates. The spermatozoa of the hydrozoan *Campanularia* orientate and swim towards the female gonangium, or alternatively follow a gradient of female gonangial extract. In the siphonophoran *Muggiaea*, the chemical attractant is produced by an extracellular structure of the oocyte called the cupule. In both cases the nature of the chemoattractants are unknown, although they appear to be low molecular weight proteins. In all other cases the encounter of gametes apparently occurs randomly. Rothschild and Swann in the early 1950s calculated the theoretical collision rate of sea urchin oocytes and spermatozoa by treating the fertilization reaction as a first order chemical reaction, i.e. they estimated the probability of a sperm–oocyte collision using parameters such as sperm density, speed of the spermatozoon and oocyte radius. The actual successful collision rate at a particular density may be determined by kinetic experiments. This method involves dropping oocytes into a freshly prepared suspension of spermatozoa and then taking aliquots at fixed time intervals, i.e. 5 seconds, 10 seconds, 30 seconds, 60 seconds, etc. A small amount of detergent, such as sodium lauryl sulphate, is added to each aliquot to immediately stop the 'fertilization reaction'. Effectively all oocytes which have already interacted with a spermatozoon continue to develop, while the fertilizing capacity of all remaining free spermatozoa is abolished.

Capacitation

Although sperm–oocyte interaction in most species, particularly those practising external fertilization, appears to be a random event, spermatozoa from many animals exhibit behavioural changes when they contact the oocyte

Table 3.1 *Time required for capacitation in different species*

Species	Time required for capacitation	Duration of sperm motility (h)	Duration of sperm fertility (h)	Fertilizable life of oocytes(h)
Mouse	<1	13	6	15
Sheep	1–5	48	30–48	12–15
Rat	2–3	17	14	12
Hamster	2–4	–	–	9–12
Pig	3–6	50	24–48	10
Rabbit	5	43–50	28–36	6–8
Rhesus monkey	5–6	–	–	23
Human	5–6	48–60	24–48	6–24
Dog	–	268	134	24

surface or female tissues. These behavioural changes, which have been termed capacitation, are essential for successful fertilization. In amphibians, spermatozoa attain the ability to fertilize following exposure to the jelly layers surrounding the oocyte, which are a product of the female reproductive tract. The frog *Discoglossus* provides an interesting example: ejaculated spermatozoa of this anuran are immotile and organized into bundles. Upon contact with the outermost jelly layer of the oocyte individual spermatozoa start moving, escape from the bundle and penetrate the gelatinous animal plug. Sperm motility in some teleost fish also seems to be enhanced when they contact the surface of the chorion, while sperm of the hydroid *Campanularia* must interact with a surface component of the gonangium epithelial cells before attaining fertilizability.

Capacitation of mammalian spermatozoa, which takes place in the female genital tract, is more fully understood. The time required for capacitation varies from species to species and ranges from less than 1 hour in the mouse to 6 hours in humans (Table 3.1). Two changes seem to occur: first the removal of epididymal and seminal plasma proteins coating the spermatozoa, followed by an alteration in the glycoproteins of the sperm plasma membranes. Capacitation may take place within the uterus or oviducts, or in vitro by contact with the cumulus oophorus. In the latter case, the spermatozoa become intimately attached to the cumulus cells for 2–3 hours, during which time these cells, by secreting glycosidases, alter the sperm surface components. Follicular fluid can also promote capacitation in vitro. A low molecular weight motility factor found in follicular fluid, ovary, uterus and oviduct may increase sperm metabolism (and hence motility) by lowering ATP and increasing cyclic AMP levels within the sperm. Table 3.1 demonstrates the duration of fertility and motility of mammalian spermatozoa within the oviduct, together with the fertilizable life of oocytes.

Activation of the oocyte and cell cycle regulation

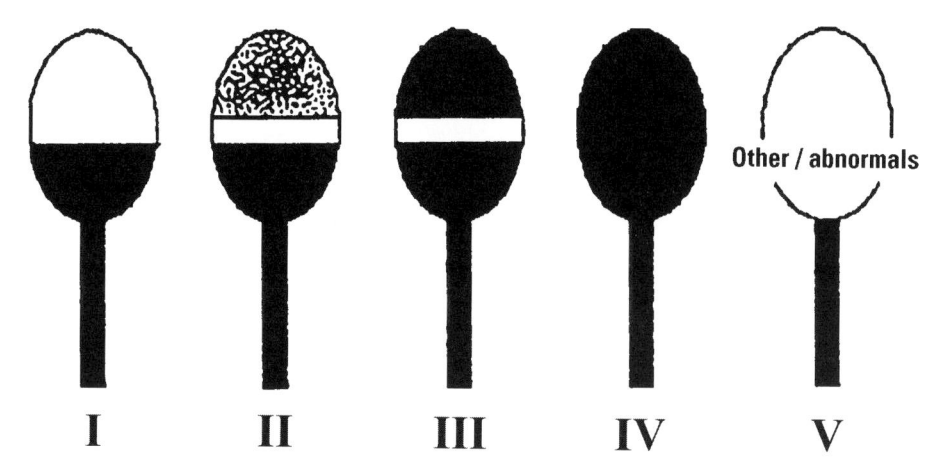

Figure 3.3 The ARIC test: a population of spermatozoa are exposed to the calcium ionophore A23187 and then labelled with fluorescent lectins for specific surface sugars. The white area indicates fluorescence. I: acrosome intact; II: incomplete acrosome reaction; III: complete acrosome reaction; IV: dead sperm; V: abnormal sperm.

Acrosome reaction

The acrosome reaction is the final prerequisite step in the activation of the spermatozoon before gamete fusion is possible. First, there is an absolute Ca^{2+} requirement: the acrosome reaction only occurs in the presence of Ca^{2+}. The reaction may also be induced artificially by adding the ionophore A23187 (Figure 3.3), a chemical which carries Ca^{2+} across cell membranes, to the sperm medium, or simply by increasing the environmental concentration of Ca^{2+}. An artificially high pH of about 9–9.5 will also induce this reaction, and it is also well known that invertebrate spermatozoa release H^+ when activated. Finally, the polymerization of sub-acrosomal actin which causes the extension of the acrosomal tubule depends on the influx of cations, particularly Mg^{2+} and K^+. Although the minute size of the male gamete hinders experimentation, it appears that the physiological events leading to the acrosome reaction parallel those leading to activation of the oocyte. These include changes in the ion permeability of the plasma membrane, alterations in the intracellular level of free Ca^{2+} and an alkalinization of the cytoplasm.

Activation of the oocyte and cell cycle regulation

There are two current hypotheses as to how a spermatozoon triggers the oocyte into metabolic activity. One school of thought proposed by Dale and his colleagues in the early 1980s suggests the presence of a soluble factor in the sper-

28 *Sperm–oocyte interaction*

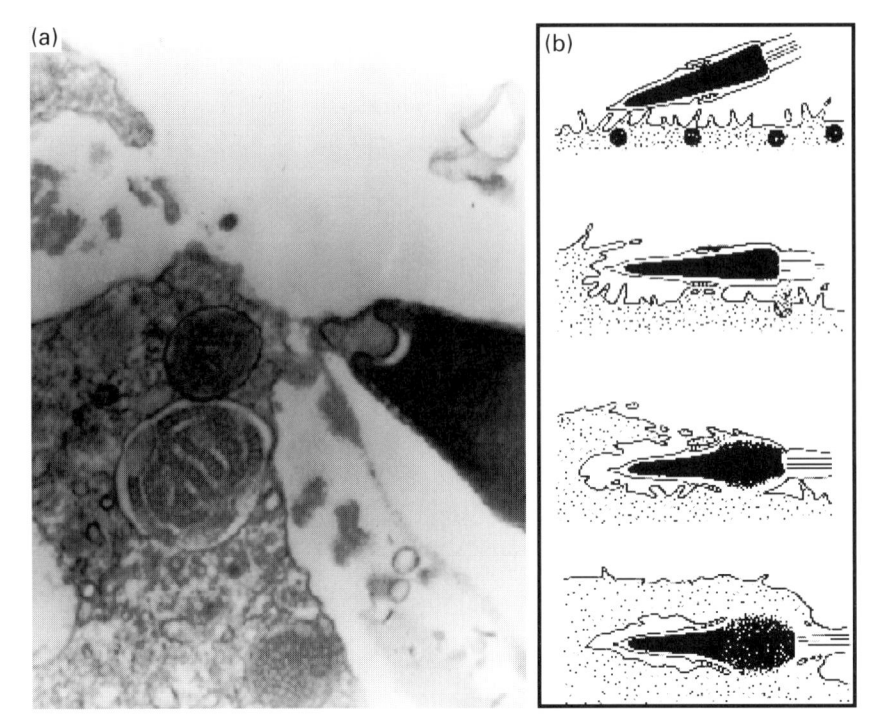

Figure 3.4 (a) Transmission electron micrograph showing the point of sperm–oocyte fusion in the sea urchin. Sperm factor must flow through this cytoplasmic bridge of 0.1 μm diameter. The large granule (1 μm) below the spermatozoon is a cortical granule. (b) Stages in sperm–oocyte fusion in the mammal. Modified from Yanagimachi (1994).

matozoon that is released into the oocyte following gamete fusion (Figure 3.4). The contrasting idea proposes that the interaction between the spermatozoon and a receptor on the oocyte surface prior to fusion is transduced to the oocyte interior via G-proteins or tyrosine kinase.

The first event of activation in most oocytes is a depolarization of the plasma membrane. One notable exception is the hamster oocyte, which appears to undergo a series of hyperpolarizations. Close observation of the electrical response in sea urchins showed it to be biphasic, with a small step-like depolarization preceding the larger fertilization potential. Later studies showed that only successful spermatozoa gave rise to this initial event and that it also occurred in ascidian and amphibian oocytes. As cortical granule exocytosis is not initiated until about the time of the second, larger depolarization, the fertilization potential, the period between the two events, corresponds approximately to what has been called the latent period. Single channel recordings, using the patch clamp technique, showed that the channels underlying the fertilization current had a conductance of 400 pS and were non-specific for ions. By measuring the total cell conductance at fertilization and the single channel conductance, and knowing the probability that a channel is in the open state, it was estimated that about 1000 fertilization channels were activated by the spermatozoon close to the site of fusion. Later work showed that the channels were not gated by intracellular Ca^{2+} but possibly by IP3. In conclusion, in invertebrate oocytes the spermatozoon induces an inward current in the oocyte plasma membrane by activating non-specific ion channels shortly following gamete fusion.

The situation in the human is quite different: the spermatozoon induces an outward current in the oocyte plasma membrane by activating potassium channels. A second difference was found in the mechanism of fertilization channel gating, where the human potassium channel is calcium gated. In the ascidian, the channel is not calcium gated (Figure 3.5).

The second activation event is a transient but massive release of calcium from intracellular stores that starts at the point of sperm–oocyte fusion and traverses the oocytes as a wave towards the antipode. Owing to the rapid succession of change in the oocyte during activation it is difficult to distinguish individual events. Using immature germinal vesicle stage sea urchin oocytes, it was shown that the preliminary step was the result of fusion. This was later confirmed by a second research group who utilized capacitance measurements to indicate confluity of the two plasma membranes. As fusion precedes activation, this gives support to the soluble sperm-borne factor hypothesis. Further support may be drawn from inter-phylum cross-fertilization where activation will only occur in the presence of fusogens. Shortly after the appearance of the fertilization potential in sea urchins and ascidians, there is a massive release of Ca^{2+} from intracellular stores that causes an increase in cytosolic Ca^{2+} from 0.1 µM to 10 µM. Within minutes the Ca^{2+} returns to resting levels. The elevated Ca^{2+} starts at the point of sperm–oocyte fusion and traverses the oocyte to the antipode in about 10 seconds. Smaller repetitive waves continue for many minutes after fertilization. The mechanism involved in wave propagation is not clear, and could be dependent on Ca^{2+}-induced Ca^{2+} release (as in muscle), or IP3–induced Ca^{2+} release. This is followed by a wave of cortical exocytosis in regulative eggs, or a surface contraction in ascidian oocytes which travels in the same direction as the calcium wave. In the hamster the Ca^{2+} wave also starts near the site of sperm attachment and spreads to the antipode within 4–7 seconds, ending 15–20 seconds later. These Ca^{2+} waves are repetitive, occurring with an interval of 3 minutes, and may be induced by microinjecting soluble sperm factors into oocytes. Repetitive calcium spikes are also seen in the

30 *Sperm–oocyte interaction*

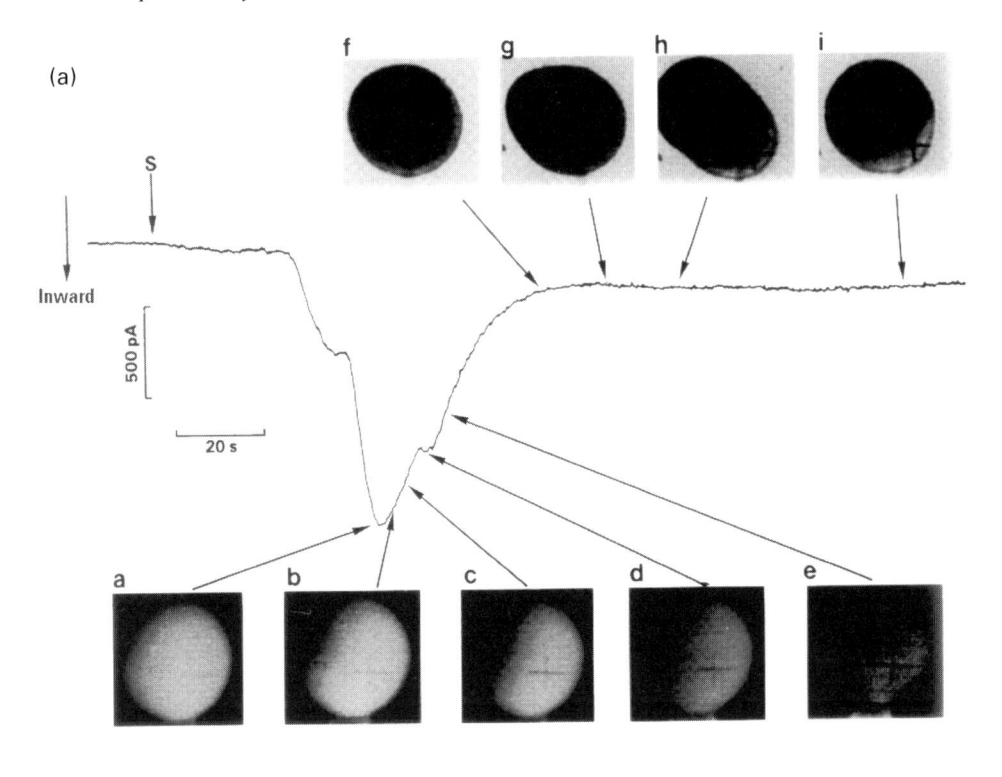

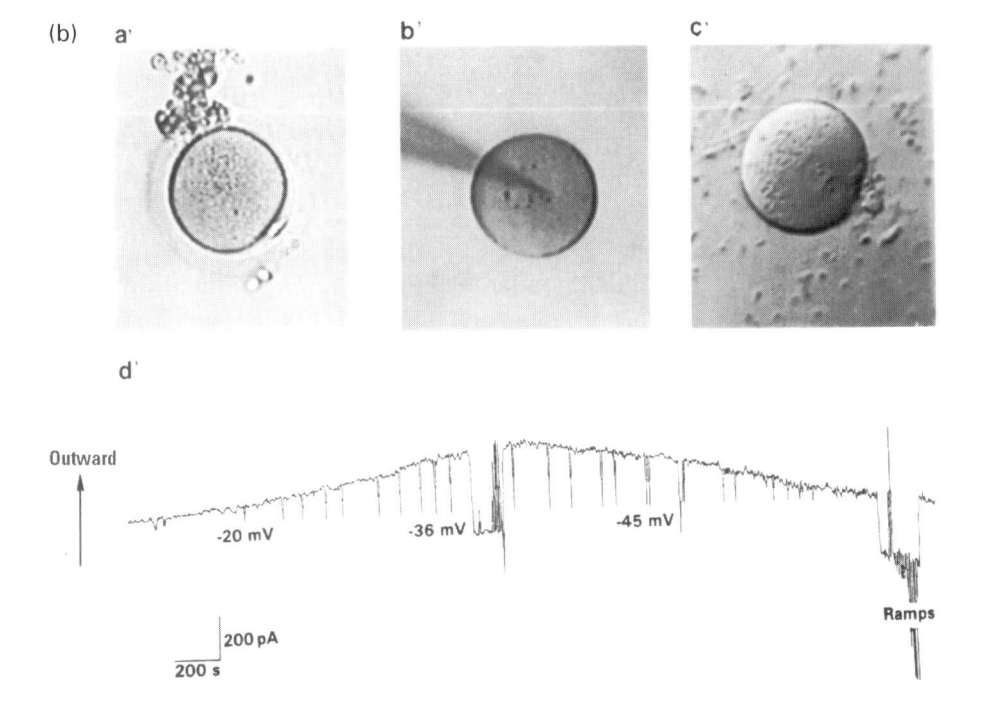

human oocyte during fertilization, or following microinjection of sperm factors or whole spermatozoa for intracytoplasmic sperm injection (ICSI). In sea urchins and amphibians the spermatozoon triggers two ionic signals: the second is an increase in intracellular pH. In sea urchins the second product of phosphoinositide hydrolysis, diacylglycerol, leads to activation of the Na^+/H^+ exchange mechanism by activating protein kinase C, causing an alkalinization of the cytoplasm. This increase in pH is necessary for several of the later events of activation. The majority of oocytes are blocked in meiotic arrest either at metaphase I or metaphase II, by the presence of high levels of maturation promoting factor (MPF) and cytostatic factor (CSF). It is thought that oocyte activation leads to CSF breakdown, cyclin degradation and hence MPF inactivation. This field of research is in continuous evolution but it seems probable that the calcium signal triggers MPF inactivation via calmodulin kinase II. Cell cycle checkpoints are shown in Figure 3.6.

The cortical reaction and structural reorganization

Oocyte structure may be modified in several ways during activation. In some oocytes there is a dramatic redistribution of cytoplasmic organelles which prepares the zygote for embryogenesis, while in others the cell surface contracts at one pole and expands at the other. Perhaps the first, and certainly the most obvious change comes about as a result of the cortical reaction. Cortical granules are found in the oocytes of many animals, for example echinoderms, some mammals, amphibians, annelids, fish and crustacea, although there is tremendous diversity in their form and size. In mammals, sea urchins and starfish they are found immediately below the plasma membrane in a single layer, whereas in some ophiuroid echinoderms (brittle stars) they are found several layers deep (Figure 3.7). These special organelles originate as vesicles in the Golgi complex and contain, amongst other substances, enzymes and mucopolysaccharides. During activation the granules break open releasing their contents into the perivitelline space (the gap between the oocyte plasma

Figure 3.5 (a) Activation events in the ascidian oocyte. The top frames (f–i) show the surface contraction, the middle trace the slow, bell-shaped inward fertilization current, and the lower frames (a–e) a wave of high intracellular calcium traversing the cell from the site of sperm entry to the antipode. (b) A physiologically competent human metaphase II oocyte with intact zona pellucida (a'), during whole-cell clamp recording (b') and following activation showing two pronuclei (c'). d' is the outward activation current in the human oocyte that is generated by the activation of calcium activated potassium channels.

32 *Sperm–oocyte interaction*

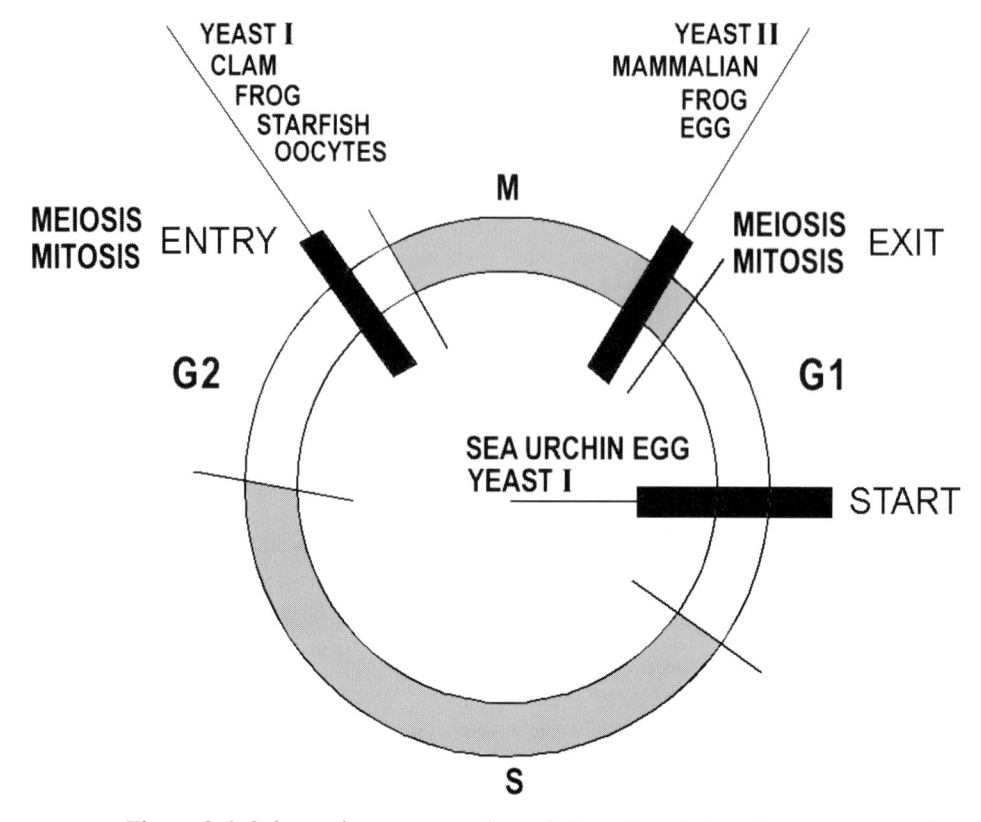

Figure 3.6 Schematic representation of the cell cycle in mitosis and meiosis showing G1, S, G2, and M phases and control points. Modified from Whittaker (1990).

membrane and the vitelline coat). There are two immediate consequences of cortical granule exocytosis: the perivitelline space first increases in volume, and the vitelline coat is then transformed into a thick, hard protective structure.

Most of our information on cortical granule exocytosis has been gained from studies on the sea urchin oocyte. There are about 20 000 cortical granules per oocyte; they are membrane bound, about 1 μm in diameter, and their contents often look star or spiral-shaped. The granules appear to be interconnected by thin filaments and are firmly attached to the oocyte surface. A tangential section through an oocyte clearly shows their homogeneous distribution just below the cell surface. Exocytosis starts some 10 seconds after the spermatozoon has attached to the vitelline coat. This delay is called the latent period. The granules in the immediate vicinity of the spermatozoon are the first to break down, and a wave of exocytosis then spreads slowly around the oocyte surface. Mucopolysaccharides, released from the granules into the perivitelline space, cause a rapid influx of water which distends the vitelline coat, lifting it

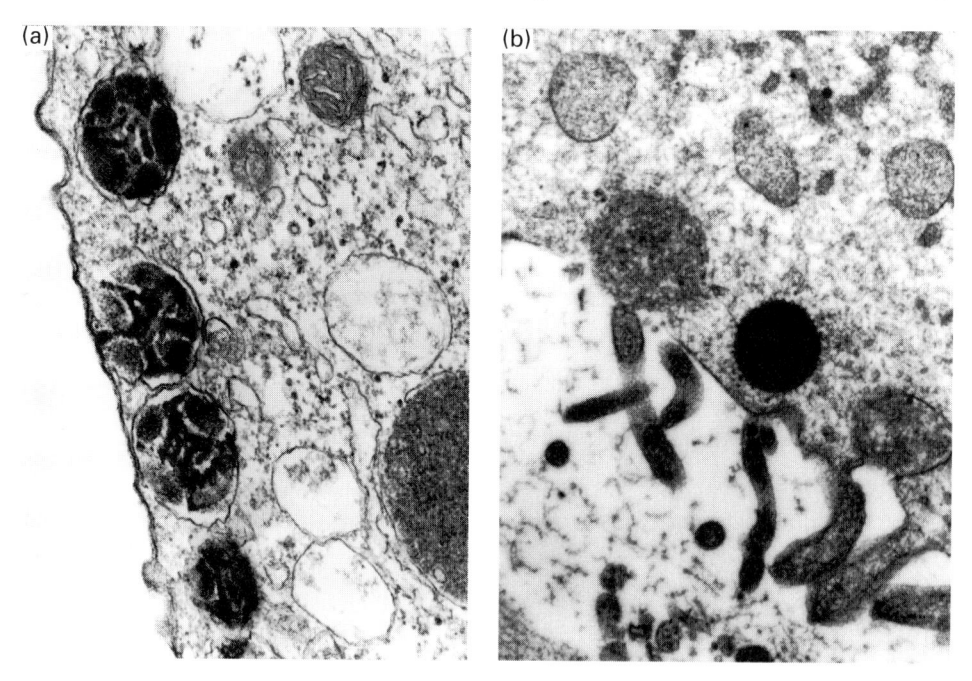

Figure 3.7 Transmission electron micrographs of the surface of unfertilized oocytes of the sea urchin (a) and human (b), showing the cortical granules.

1–20 μm away from the oocyte surface. This wavelike progression of cortical granule exocytosis and the concomitant elevation of the vitelline coat takes approximately 20 seconds to spread around the oocyte surface. Over the next 5 minutes the perivitelline space continues to increase and the vitelline coat hardens and thickens becoming the familiar fertilization membrane. Although it is not clear how the cortical reaction is initiated, or how it is propagated around the oocyte, an important factor is the increase in cytoplasmic Ca^{2+}. Cortical granule exocytosis may be induced by injecting Ca^{2+} into the cytoplasm, and it can be prevented using Ca^{2+} chelating agents (molecules which bind free Ca^{2+}). Furthermore, oocytes exposed to ionophores (molecules which facilitate the passage of ions across membranes) such as amphotericin B or A23187 undergo the cortical reaction along with several other activation events. Finally, it should be pointed out that cortical granule exocytosis is essentially a process of membrane fusion, and each granule fuses with the inner aspect of the plasma membrane. In order to fuse, the granules must come into close contact with the oocyte surface and it appears that the cytoskeleton is involved in this movement. The oocyte plasma membrane becomes a mosaic structure made up of the original membrane and the incorporated patches of cortical granules. The physiological characteristics of these inserted patches of new membrane is not known, nor is it known whether they are essential for embryogenesis; however, they do cause a considerable increase in the surface area of the oocyte.

What about the more obvious structural modifications resulting from the cortical reaction? The vitelline coat of the unfertilized oocyte is a fibrous glycoprotein structure approximately 15 nm thick. Immediately following elevation it remains thin and elastic and can easily be digested by proteolytic enzymes. During the next 5 minutes it becomes thicker, reaching approximately 90 nm, and much harder. The fertilization membrane is a laminar structure, and it is thought that the crystalline component of the cortical granules attaches to the inner aspect of the vitelline coat thereby thickening it. A trypsin-like protease also released from the granules plays an important role in this thickening and hardening; if this protease is specifically inhibited the fertilization membrane fails to harden. A further component of the granules is a calcium-binding glycoprotein which tightly adheres to the oocyte surface forming the hyaline layer. In actual fact, a very thin hyaline layer may be present before fertilization (also of cortical granule origin) which then thickens as a result of the cortical reaction.

Teleost fish oocytes have cortical alveoli which also break down in a wavelike progression from the point of sperm entry, releasing their contents into the perivitelline space. A hyaline layer is formed, the chorion hardens and water enters into the perivitelline space causing it to increase in volume. In contrast to the situation in the sea urchin the perivitelline space swells not by distension of the chorion (vitelline coat) but by shrinkage of the oocyte surface. The cortical alveoli of the marine worm *Nereis* also break down in a wave-like fashion during activation and, similar to the situation in fish, the perivitelline space increases by oocyte shrinkage rather than by membrane elevation. A peculiar observation is that the alveolar contents extrude outside the oocyte surface layers and by hydration form a thick impervious jelly-like structure. Some mammalian oocytes also contain cortical granules which upon activation break open releasing their contents; the zona pellucida hardens and thickens, and this is known as the zona reaction.

In some amphibians cortical granule exocytosis and elevation of the vitelline coat is remarkably similar to that in the sea urchin. The jelly layer apparently plays a different role in these two groups of animal. In the sea urchin the jelly layer, now on the outside of the fertilization membrane, quickly dissolves. In the frog the jelly layer swells immensely after fertilization and serves (1) for protection, (2) to allow the oocytes to attach to submerged structures, and (3) to keep oocytes spaced and thus allow them enough room for metabolic turnover with the environment. Even in oocytes which lack cortical granules, such as those of the ascidian, there appears to be some sort of exocytosis of cortical material at activation and, in some species at least, the perivitelline space expands. In ascidians changes in permeability to ions and other molecules provide evidence that the plasma membrane is also reorganized.

The role of cortical reorganization

Cortical reorganization is a common feature of oocyte activation. Although mechanisms differ, the results are often similar. The sea urchin oocyte has been studied in great detail, other oocytes less so. By piecing together all the information some general conclusions may be drawn regarding the role of cortical re-organization in embryogenesis. First and foremost the developing embryo must be protected in some way. In oocytes which lack cortical granules, for example those of ascidians and insects, a protective structure which does not alter much following activation is laid down during oogenesis – i.e. it is preformed. In other animals a different strategy is employed. The oocyte has a relatively thin extracellular coat which hardens after activation, catalysed by the cortical granule products. In either event the embryo remains in its protective coat until hatching. A second extracellular structure produced as a result of cortical granule exocytosis is the hyaline layer which serves to keep the dividing blastomeres of the embryo in close contact. The early embryo is a compact mass of continually dividing cells, and the embryo is therefore continually changing shape. Such movement would be hindered if the cells were attached to a rigid structure, so possibly for this reason the embryo is surrounded by the fluid-filled perivitelline space. This gap may also serve as a micro-environment buffering the embryo from changes in the environment.

Reorganization of the plasma membrane appears to be related to the metabolic de-repression of the oocyte and occurs both in oocytes with, and those without, cortical granules. Certainly, this reorganization is dramatic and rapid in granule-containing oocytes and is attained without the participation of the cells' synthetic apparatus. Although we do not know the function of this mosaic plasma membrane, the resulting transient increase in surface area will facilitate the metabolic turnover of the activated oocyte. Finally, the cortical changes will exclude the interaction of supernumerary spermatozoa within a limited range of sperm density and in fact many authors have suggested that such changes have evolved specifically as polyspermy-preventing mechanisms; however, perhaps one should be more objective. Certainly in some animals, for example mammals, insects and nematodes, the sperm:oocyte ratio is so low under natural conditions that supernumerary collisions are extremely unlikely and therefore cortical changes may well have other functions, mobilized by the increase in intracellular Ca^{2+}.

Events leading to the formation of the zygote nucleus

In marine invertebrates, the tip of the acrosomal tubule makes contact with and then fuses with the oocyte plasma membrane. In mammals, where there is no acrosomal tubule, the spermatozoal plasma membrane in the post-acrosomal region fuses with the oocyte plasma membrane; by fusion we mean that the two membranes become continuous The process of membrane fusion between gametes (or for that matter somatic cells) is not understood, but Ca^{2+} and a close approximation of the two membranes is essential. Fusion of gametes seems to be facilitated by the presence of numerous microvilli on the oocyte surface (Figure 3.8); these have a low radius of curvature which may help to overcome opposing electrostatic charges. In fact, spermatozoa rarely fuse with the microvillus-free areas of the oocyte surface, for example the area over the second metaphase spindle of mouse oocytes. During fusion the oocyte cytoplasm rises up in a protuberance around the spermatozoal nucleus to form the fertilization cone. In the sea urchin, microfilaments appear to be involved in the formation and resorption of this structure.

It would be interesting to know if some of the enzymes released from the acrosome alter the oocyte plasma membrane, preparing it for the subsequent fusion process. One possibility is that the release of phospholipases and the transient production of lysophospholipids destabilizes the plasma membrane by altering the normal phospholipid components. In mammals and sea urchins, the fertilizing spermatozoon continues flagellar movement for some 20 seconds after attachment to the oocyte surface. There then follows a sudden cessation of flagellar motion, which may occur simultaneously with the process of gamete fusion. In the sea urchin the spermatozoal tail becomes erect and perpendicular to the oocyte surface. The fertilization membrane elevates around the tail and, during the next 30 seconds the fertilization cone develops and the spermatozoon moves into the oocyte at a rate of 5 μm/s. Once in the cortex, the naked spermatozoal nucleus moves laterally, rotates approximately 180 degrees and during the next 10 minutes develops into the male pronucleus. The mitochondria and tail of the spermatozoon also enter the cytoplasm but later degenerate.

The process in small mammals is somewhat slower; sperm–oocyte fusion is quite advanced after 3 minutes, the entire incorporation of the spermatozoal head takes 15 minutes, and pronucleus formation takes about 60 minutes. In

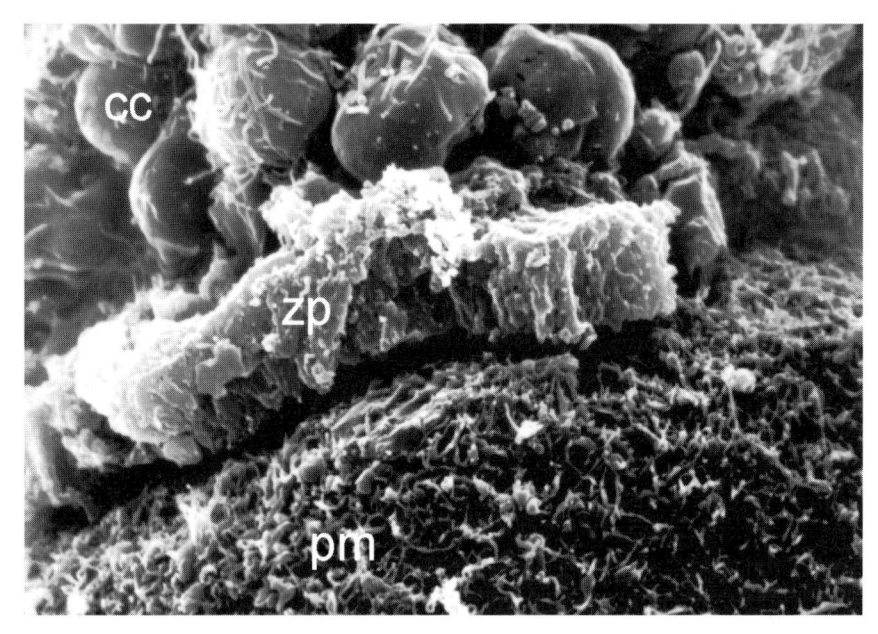

Figure 3.8 Scanning electron micrograph of the surface of an unfertilized metaphase II human oocyte, with the zona pellucida (zp) and cumulus cells (cc) partially dissected to demonstrate the microvillar organization of the plasma membrane.

some mammals (for example Chinese hamster) the tail is not incorporated, while in others it is incorporated by the progressive fusion of the oocyte and spermatozoal plasma membranes. After incorporation, the middle-piece mitochondria and axial filament of the tail appear to disintegrate. The spermatozoal plasma membrane, however, is integrated into the oocyte plasma membrane and may play a role in development.

The formation and fusion of the pronuclei

Transformation of the spermatozoal nucleus into the male pronucleus involves chromatin dispersion, nuclear enlargement, the disintegration of the nuclear envelope and the formation of a new pronuclear envelope. The spermatozoal nuclear membrane breaks down by the formation of multiple fusions between the inner and outer laminae; this develops into a loose array of vesicles around the now dispersed chromatin. Formation of the new envelope is essentially the reverse of this process; vesicles aggregate at the periphery of the dispersed chromatin, fuse, and form a typical porous nuclear envelope. Male pronucleus development requires specific cytoplasmic conditions which are found in the mature oocyte, but not in the immature oocyte (germinal vesicle stage). A male pronucleus growth factor has been proposed; this may be a disulphide-reducing agent, as the sperm chromatin of some mammals is maintained in a condensed state partly by disulphide cross-linkage of the nucleohistones. Alternatively, the cytoplasmic conditions required for male pronuclear development may be multiple.

In oocytes which are normally fertilized before the completion of meiosis, de-condensation of the sperm chromatin has to await the ejection of the second polar body. The female pronucleus may either be already formed, as in sea urchins and coelenterates, or alternatively develops following sperm entry and the completion of meiosis. In mammals, the haploid female chromosomes start to disperse, vesicles form around them and fuse to form a bilaminar envelope. The male and female pronuclei now migrate towards each other and subsequently move towards the centre of the oocyte; the sperm aster appears to be involved in this movement. In sea urchins, the envelopes of the two pronuclei fuse to form a zygote nuclear envelope, containing the decondensed male and female chromatin. In most other animals (and as originally described for *Ascaris* by E.B. Wilson), the chromosomes in each pronucleus condense and concomitantly the pronuclear envelopes break down without fusing together. The male and female chromosomes then intermix in the cytoplasm and form the metaphase of the first mitotic spindle (Figure 3.9).

Sperm–oocyte interaction in mammals

In mammals, fertilization is internal and the male gametes must be introduced into the female tract at coitus. Coitus itself ranges from minutes in humans to hours in camels but is accompanied by many physiological changes. Penile erection in humans may be elicited by tactile and psychogenic stimuli such as visual cues. A decrease in resistance and consequently dilatation in the arteries supplying the penis with closure of the arteriovenous shunts and venous bleed valves causes erection. The testes may increase their volume by as much as 50% owing to vasocongestion. Ejaculation of semen is achieved by contraction of the smooth muscles of the urethra and the striated muscles in the penis. Muscle contraction is sequential and results in the mixing of the prostatic liquid rich in acid phosphatase, the vas deferens fraction containing spermatozoa, and the seminal vesicle fraction containing fructose.

In the woman tactile stimulation of the glans clitoris and vaginal wall leads to engorgement of the vagina and labia majora and an increase in vaginal dimension. At orgasm, frequent vaginal contractions occur, and uterine contractions begin in the fundus and spread to the lower uterine segment. In humans, rabbit,

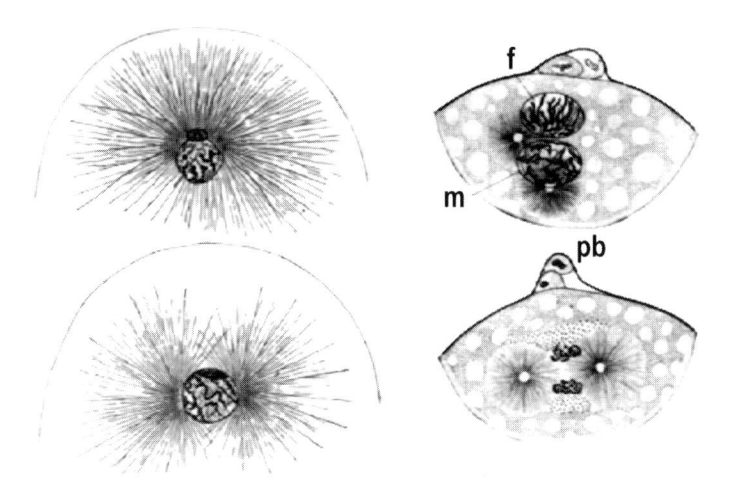

Figure 3.9 A drawing from Wilson (1900) showing (left) the fusion of male and female pronuclei to form the zygote nucleus as in sea urchins. In the majority of animals (and usually in mammals) the pronuclear membranes break down without fusing, allowing the chromosomes to interact in the cytoplasm (frames on the right).

sheep, cow and cat the semen is ejaculated into the vagina. In the pig, dog and horse it is deposited directly into the cervix and uterus. In many species the semen coagulates rapidly after deposition in the female tract, as a result of interaction with an enzyme of prostatic origin. The coagulation may serve to retain spermatozoa in the vagina or to protect them from the acid environment. In the human, this coagulation is dissolved within 1 hour by progressive action of a second pro-enzyme, also of prostatic origin. Within minutes of mating spermatozoa may be detected in the cervix or uterus. In the human 99% of the spermatozoa are lost from the vagina. The few that enter the tract may survive for many hours in the cervical crypts of mucus. In the absence of progesterone, cervical mucus permits sperm penetration into the upper female tract.

Although data is inconclusive it appears that activity of the musculature of the female tract is not required for sperm transport. Prostaglandins present in the semen are also not required for sperm transport, as these are removed in artificial insemination. It is probable that the spermatozoa move through the uterus under their own propulsion and are transported in currents set up by the action of uterine cilia. The cervical crypts may serve as a reservoir regulating flow of spermatozoa into the tract, while the utero–tubal junction may act as a sphincter. The earliest appearance of spermatozoa in the oviducts is 4–7 hours in hamster and rabbit. Few sperm reach the ampullae and in the mouse sperm–oocyte ratios in the ampullae are usually 1:1.

Before gaining the ability to fertilize oocytes, ejaculated mammalian spermatozoa must reside a minimum period in the female reproductive tract. This relatively undefined process, called capacitation, is thought to involve the removal of glycoproteins from the sperm surface exposing receptor sites that can respond to oocyte signals and lead to the acrosome reaction. As epididymal maturation and capacitation are unique to mammals, this may represent an evolutionary adaptation to internal fertilization. In the human, capacitation probably starts while the spermatozoa are passing through the cervix. Many enzymes and factors from the female tract have been implicated in causing capacitation, such as arylsulphatase, fucosidase and taurine; however, to date the precise mechanism remains unknown. Certainly the factors are not species specific, and capacitation may be induced in vitro in the absence of female signals. Capacitation is temperature dependent and only occurs at 37–39 °C. Sperm surface components are removed or altered during capacitation. For example, an antigen on the plasma membrane of the mouse spermatozoon, laid down during epididymal maturation, cannot be removed by repeated washing, but disappears, or is masked during capacitation.

The acrosome is a membrane-bound cap covering the anterior portion of the sperm head and is found in the majority of species (Figure 3.10). This structure, or its surrounding membranes, contains a large array of hydrolytic enzymes including hyaluronidase, acrosin, proacrosin, phosphatase, arylsuphatase, collagenase, phospholipase C and beta-galactosidase, to mention a few. The acrosome reaction involves fusion of the outer acrosomal membrane with the overlying plasma membrane allowing the acrosomal contents to be released. In the human, fusion appears to take place initially near the border of the acrosomal cap region and the equatorial segment of the acrosome. The acrosome reaction is relatively rapid once the correct trigger signals have been received and may take from 2–15 minutes in vitro. Gametes collected from the ampullae of mammals after mating show that, while free swimming spermatozoa have unreacted acrosomes, those within the cumulus mass have either reacted acrosomes, or are in the process of reacting. The majority of spermatozoa attached to the surface of the zona pellucida surface have reacted acrosomes. One of the glycoproteins of the mouse zona pellucida, ZP3, binds to the plasma membrane over the acrosomal cap and induces the acrosome reaction. It is not clear whether the acrosome reaction is initiated while the spermatozoon is interacting with the cumulus mass. A major component of the cumulus matrix is hyaluronic acid, and as the acrosome contains hyaluronidase, it is feasible to suggest that the reaction may start in the cumulus. Whatever the natural signal for induction, the acrosome reaction may also be induced in vitro in the absence of any maternal signal. In mammalian spermatozoa ZP3 may be con-

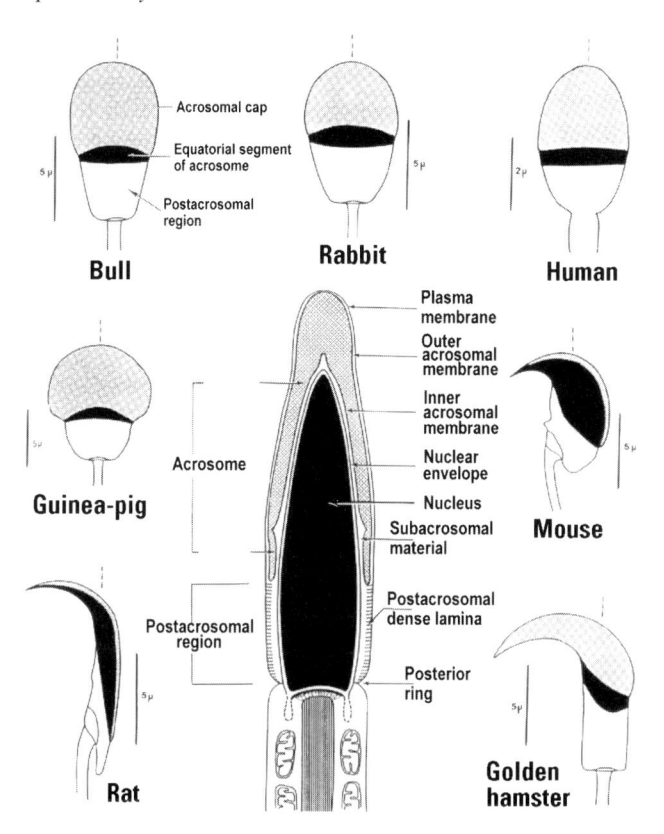

Figure 3.10 Variation in shape of mammalian spermatozoa with, at the centre, a schematic representation showing the layout of the several membranes. Modified from Yanagimachi (1994).

sidered a regulatory ligand which triggers the acrosome reaction. G-proteins are found in the plasma membrane and outer acrosomal membranes.

Although we are far from understanding the sequence of events leading to exocytosis, potential second messenger pathways involved include adenylate cyclase generating cAMP, phospholipase C generating InsP3 and diacylglycerol (DAG), phospholipase D generating phosphatidic acid, and Phospholipase A_2 generating arachidonic acid. Completion of the acrosome reaction does not necessarily ensure the success of in vitro fertilization. In a population of spermatozoa surrounding the cumulus mass we may expect enormous variability. Some will acrosome react too soon, others too late; in some the trigger stimulus will be inadequate, perhaps in others the transduction mechanism will fail at some point. The cumulus mass is composed of both cellular and acellular components. The acellular matrix is made up of proteins and carboyhydrates, including hyaluronic acid. In vivo very few spermatozoa reach the site of fertilization: therefore the idea derived from in vitro fertilization studies, that large populations of spermatozoa surrounding the oocyte mass dissolve the cumulus matrix is probably incorrect in vivo. Fertilization occurs before the dispersion of the cumulus mass, and in vivo the sperm:oocyte ratio is close to 1:1.

The zona pellucida, a glycoprotein sheet several microns thick secreted by the growing oocyte, has a chemical composition which consists of 70%, protein, 20% hexose, 3% sialic acid and 2% sulphate. Electron microscopy shows the outer surface to have a latticed appearance. There are three major glycoproteins known as ZPl, ZP2, and ZP3, whose distribution in the human zona remains unknown at present. In the mouse ZP2 is distributed throughout the thickness of the zona. Spermatozoa penetrate the zona in 2–15 minutes, and sperm binding to the mouse zona is mediated by the ZP3 glycoprotein. The exact nature of the complementary receptor molecule on the surface of the spermatozoon is not known, and may be either protein or glycoprotein. In the mouse, the sperm receptors appear to be on the surface of the plasma membrane of the acrosome intact spermatozoon. Receptors for ZP2, in contrast, are located on the inner acrosomal membrane and therefore are unmasked after the acrosome reaction. According to Wassarman and colleagues sperm-receptor activity resides in the O-linked oligosaccharides of ZP3. The complementary molecule of the spermatozoon may be a lectin-like protein. It has been suggested, both in invertebrates and in mammals, that sperm binding to its receptor on the zona is an enzyme–substrate interaction. During penetration of the zona the spermatozoon loses its acrosomal contents and only the inner acrosomal membrane is in direct contact with the zona. While passing through the zona the spermatozoon beats its tail strongly leaving a sharp pathway behind. In eutherian mammals, the sperm-head plasma membrane of the postacrosomal region apparently fuses with the oocyte plasma membrane; however, this region of the plasma membrane only attains fusibility after the acrosome reaction. The surface of most oocytes, including the human oocyte, is organized into evenly spaced short microvilli. In mouse and hamster the area overlying the metaphase spindle is microvillus-free and spermatozoa are incapable or less likely to fuse with this area. The human oocyte is an exception, having no obvious surface polarity, with microvilli present over the entire surface from the animal pole to the vegetal pole.

Following gamete fusion the sperm plasma membrane remains in the oocyte plasma membrane and indicates the point of fusion. In the rat, a fluorescently-labelled conjugated antibody to a sperm plasma membrane antigen shows that immediately after fusion the sperm plasma membrane remains localized to the point of entry and by the pronucleate stage the antigen spreads all over the surface of the zygote. Sperm motility, although necessary for penetration of the zona, is not required for gamete fusion. Fusion is temperature, pH and Ca^{2+} dependent. As fusion of spermatozoa to nude oocytes is not inhibited in the presence of monosaccharides or lectins, it seems that the terminal saccharides of glycoproteins are not directly involved in the process. Fusion of artificial membranes in apposition made of pure phospholipids has been observed experimentally, but in biological systems it appears to be mediated or facilitated by membrane associated proteins. In the guinea pig, fusion is regulated by an integral membrane protein on the posterior portion of the sperm head composed of two distinct subunits.

Shortly after gamete fusion there is a change in conductance of the oocyte plasma membrane which in mammals leads to a hyperpolarization. Shortly after detection of the fertilization potential there is a massive release of Ca^{2+} from intracellular stores, causing an increase in cytosolic Ca^{2+} from 0.1 μM to 10 μM. Within minutes the Ca^{2+} returns to resting levels. The area of Ca^{2+} elevation starts at the point of sperm–oocyte fusion and traverses the oocyte to the antipode, with smaller repetitive waves continuing many minutes after fertilization. The mechanism for wave propagation is not clear and could be either Ca^{2+}-induced Ca^{2+} release, as in muscle, or InsP3-induced Ca^{2+} release. In the hamster the Ca^{2+} wave spreads to the antipode within 4–7 seconds, ending 15–20 seconds later. These Ca^{2+} waves are repetitive, occurring with an interval of 3 minutes, and may be induced by microinjecting soluble sperm factors into oocytes.

The first morphological indication of activation in regulative oocytes is the exocytosis of cortical granules, which are small spherical membrane-bound organelles containing enzymes and mucopolysaccharides, originating as vesicles in the Golgi complex. The cortical reaction in the mammalian oocyte elicits the zona reaction, changing the characteristics of the zona pellucida. A second result of the cortical reaction is that the oocyte plasma membrane now becomes a mosaic of cortical granule membrane and the original plasma membrane. It has long been suggested that the fertilizing spermatozoon, by triggering events such as the cortical reaction, not only activates the oocyte but at the same time prevents the interaction of supernumerary spermatozoa. Certainly the alteration to the zona pellucida in the mouse, involving proteinases or glycosidases, causes a zona block with hydrolysis of ZP3 receptors which prevents them from further interaction. The mosaic zygote plasma membrane is also refractory to sperm in many species: this is known as the vitelline block. The appearance of supernumerary spermatozoa in the perivitelline space, for example in the rabbit, has been inferred to indicate a weak zona reaction and a strong vitelline reaction. In contrast, because perivitelline sperm are rare in rat, mouse, sheep and human oocytes these species were considered to have a strong zona reaction.

If we accept the premises that all spermatozoa which reach the oocyte are equally capable of fertilization, and that all areas of the oocyte surface and its extracellular coats are capable of activating spermatozoa, then the cortical reaction is too slow to be considered a block to polyspermy. The cortical reaction may serve to chemically alter the zona pellucida in order to provide a bacterially safe environment for the developing embryo. The fact that only one spermatozoon normally enters the oocyte during in vitro conditions suggests that there is a heterogeneous sperm population, and that there may be restricted areas on the oocyte surface (hot spots) for sperm entry.

During spermatogenesis the sperm nucleus is packed with distinct histones or protamines. The association of nuclear DNA with these highly charged basic amino acids is thought to cause condensation and repression of DNA activity. The rigidity of the mammalian sperm head, necessary for penetration of the zona, is due to extensive disulphide linkages in these protamines. Protamine crosslinking in the human spermatozoon is regulated by Zn^{2+} from the prostrate gland. On entering the oocyte cytoplasm the sperm nuclear envelope breaks down, the protamines are lost and pronuclear decondensation occurs. A reduced form of glutathione may be responsible for sperm nucleus decondensation. Sperm nucleus decondensing factors seem to be non-species-specific, as human sperm may decondense when microinected into amphibian oocytes.

The next step after decondensation is the formation of a new nuclear membrane around the decondensed male and female chromatin to produce the pronuclei. During pronuclear development DNA synthesis and RNA transcription occurs. Sperm pronucleus development factors are found in limited quantities within the cytoplasm, for example in the hamster a maximum of five pronuclei will decondense at any time. Again the factors are not species-specific, because human spermatozoa can develop into normal pronuclei in hamster oocytes and form a normal chromosome complement. The migration of the male and female pronuclei to the centre of the oocyte has been studied extensively, particularly in the sea urchin and the mouse. In the mouse, fluorescein conjugated probes for cytoskeletal elements show a thickened area of microfilaments below the cortex of the polar body region. In addition to the spindle microtubules there are 16 cytoplasmic microtubule organizing centres or foci. Each centrosomal focus organizes an aster. Shortly before the nuclear envelopes disintegrate the foci condense on the surface of the nuclear envelope and the first cleavage ensues. Although centrosomes are apparently inherited maternally in the mouse, in the majority of animals, including the human, centrosome inheritance is paternal.

Further reading

Dale, B. & Monroy, A. (1981) How is polyspermy prevented? *Gamete Research* 4: 151–169.

Dale, B. & Defelice, L.J. (1990) Soluble sperm factors, electrical events and egg activation. In: (Dale, B. ed.), *Mechanism of Fertilization: Plants to Humans.* Springer, Berlin, Heidelberg, New York (NATO ASI cell biology ser H 45).

Edwards, R. (1982) *Conception in the Human Female.* Academic Press, New York.

Gianaroli, L., Tosti, E., Magli, C., Ferrarreti, A. & Dale, B. (1994) The fertilization current in the human oocyte. *Molecular Reproduction Development* **38**: 209–214

Gwatkin, R. (1974) *Fertilization Mechanisms in Man and Mammals.* Plenum Press, New York.

Jaffe, L. (1980) Calcium explosions as triggers of development. *Annals of the New York Academy of Science of the USA* **339**: 86–101

Nuccitelli, R., Cherr G. & Clark, A. (1989) *Mechanisms of Egg Activation.* Plenum Press, New York.

Tesarik, I., Sousa, M. & Testart, J. (1994) Human oocyte activation after intracytoplasmic sperm injection. *Human Reproduction* **9**: 511–514.

Wassarman, P.M., Florman, H.M.& Greve, I.M. (1985) Receptor-mediated sperm-egg interactions in mammals. In: (Metz, C.B. & Monroy, A. eds), *Fertilization*, vol 2. Academic Press, New York, pp. 341–360

Wilson, E.B. (1900) *The Cell in Development and Inheritance.* Macmillan, London.

Yanagimachi, R. (1981) Mechanisms of fertilization in mammals. In: Mastroianni, L. Biggers, J.D. eds), *Fertilization and embryonic development in vitro.* Plenum Press, New York, pp. 81–182.

Yanagimachi, R. (1994) Mammalian fertilization. In: (Kuobil, E. & Neill, J., eds), *The Physiology of Reproduction.* Raven Press, New York.

4
First stages of development

After fertilization the zygote divides by mitosis into a number of smaller cells called blastomeres. This process of division, known as cleavage, is in a sense the opposite of the process of oogenesis: cleavage is a period of intense DNA replication and cell division in the absence of growth, whereas oogenesis is a period of growth without replication or division. Early cleavages are often synchronous, but sooner or later synchrony is lost. The blastomeres become organized in layers or groups, each group having a characteristic rate of cleavage. Although cleavage may be considered a mitotic process as found in adult somatic tissues there is one important difference: in adult tissue the daughter cells grow following each division and are not able to divide again until they have achieved the original size of the parent cell. The cells in a somatic population thus maintain an average size. During cleavage this is not the case: with each division the resulting blastomeres are approximately half the size of the parent blastomere. As cleavage progresses, differences arise between the blastomeres. Such differences may result from the unequal distribution of cytoplasmic components as already laid down in the oocyte during oogenesis, or from changes occurring in the blastomeres during development. Each blastomere nucleus will be subjected to a different cytoplasmic environment which in turn may differentially influence the genome activity. As a result, each blastomere sets off on its own particular programme of development and will give rise to a particular cell line, for example nerve, muscle, etc. Before discussing this phenomenon of cytoplasmic segregation and differential gene expression some examples of cleavage patterns will be considered.

Cleavage patterns

The first cleavage plane in sea urchin embryos is (as in most animals) vertical, extending from the animal to the vegetal pole. The second division is also along

Cleavage patterns 47

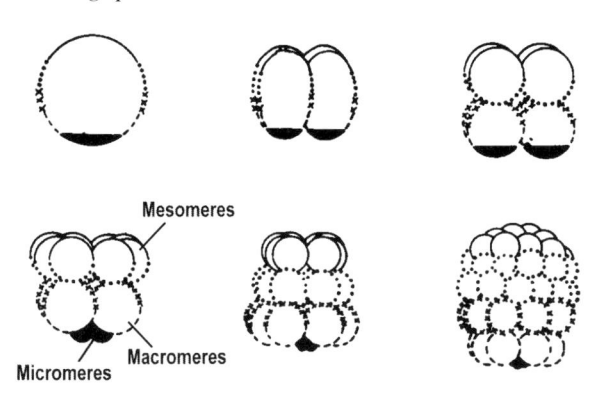

Figure 4.1 Schematic formation of the tier structure of differentiated cells in the regulative sea urchin embryo. Modified after Horstadius (1939).

the animal–vegetal (A–V) axis, but at right angles to the first. Thus at this stage there are four elongated blastomeres lying side by side (Figure 4.1). The third cleavage plane is equatorial (i.e. perpendicular to the first two planes) and divides the embryo into a tier of four animal blastomeres and a tier of four vegetal blastomeres. From now on the animal blastomeres cleave at one rate, the vegetal blastomeres at a different rate, and the blastomeres start to differ in size. The four animal blastomeres divide meridionally forming a ring of eight mesomeres, while the four vegetal blastomeres cleave horizontally with the cleavage plane shifted towards the vegetal pole. This latter division gives rise to four large macromeres and four tiny micromeres. Division continues, with the blastomeres becoming smaller and smaller until the embryo assumes a spherical shape, the blastula, consisting of a single layer of cells surrounding a liquid filled cavity, the blastocoel. The segregation of the four micromeres is of particular interest: these cells are committed to form the skeleton of the pluteus larva, and they also play an organizing role in embryogenesis.

Spiral cleavage, encountered in the molluscs, annelids and nemerteans, is similar to the above pattern; however, the mitotic spindles are positioned obliquely with respect to the axis and equator of the blastomeres and as a consequence the daughter blastomeres do not lie directly above one another. For example, consider the third cleavage in the mollusc *Trochus*. Each of the four blastomeres divides into a small micromere and a large macromere. Thus, there is an upper tier of four micromeres (animal pole) and a lower tier of four macromeres (vegetal pole). The quartet of micromeres is however shifted clockwise with respect to the macromeres so that the micromeres lie at the junctions of the lower cells rather than directly over them. Cleavage progresses in this elegant fashion forming spirals of blastomeres until late in development when the pattern becomes modified into one of bilateral symmetry.

Large quantities of yolk tend to slow down the process of cleavage and consequently the pattern of cleavage is extensively modified in yolk-rich oocytes. In amphibian oocytes the yolk is distributed in a gradient with a maximum at the vegetal pole. Cleavage in these oocytes progresses faster at the animal pole than at the vegetal pole and consequently the animal blastomeres increase in number and decrease in size at a faster rate than the vegetal blastomeres.

In all the previous examples cleavage is complete or holoblastic, dividing the entire oocyte into a number of small cells. In fish, birds and reptiles cleavages are incomplete or meroblastic, i.e. they pass through the restricted mass of cytoplasm located at the animal pole and not through the yolk. The embryo develops as a disc of cells perched on top of a yolk mass, the blastodisc. Another type of incomplete cleavage is found in the oocytes of insects. Here the zygote nucleus, lying in the centre of the oocyte, divides several times without the partitioning of the cytoplasm and the resulting nuclei migrate to the cell periphery. The peripheral cytoplasm segments around each nucleus and forms cells which remain in cytoplasmic contact with the central yolk body.

Cytoplasmic segregation and the formation of cell lines

In the previous section we looked briefly at some of the patterns of cleavage found in the animal kingdom. In some cases the pattern seems to be related to the constitution of the oocyte as laid down during oogenesis, in particular to the amount and distribution of yolk; in other cases factors controlling the positioning of the mitotic spindles seem to be important. Whichever pattern is employed, cleavage causes a partitioning of cytoplasmic components and this leads to differences in the developmental behaviour of blastomeres and the formation of different cell lines. Consider two classical examples, both marine invertebrate embryos, but quite different in their behaviour.

1. Shortly after fertilization the cytoplasmic components of the ascidian oocyte are redistributed according to a certain pattern and form five distinct territories or plasms (Figure 4.2). During cleavage these plasms become compartmentalized into different blastomeres which in turn give rise to the various cell lines. The first cleavage plane coincides with the A–V axis and divides these plasms equally between the first two blastomeres; in this way the future plane of bilateral symmetry of the larva is established. The left blastomere is committed to become the left half of the larva, the right blastomere to become the right half. Due to the small number of cells in these embryos it is relatively easy to follow cell lineage from the early cleavage stages. Each plasm gives rise to a particular tissue. For example, the yellow crescent becomes the vegetal poste-

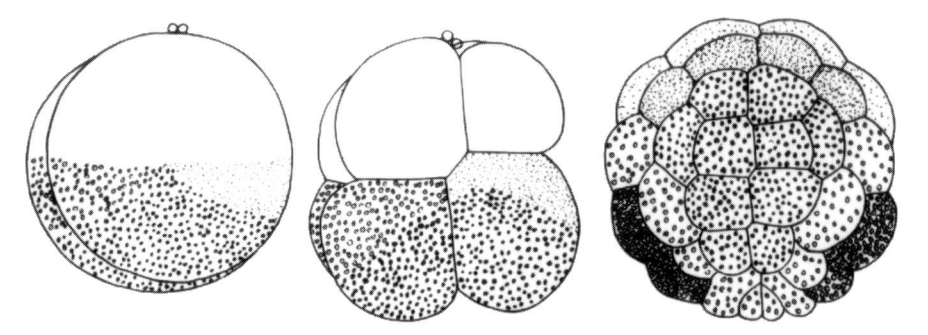

Figure 4.2 In the ascidian embryo segregation of cytoplasmic components generates different plasms that eventually localize to specific groups of cells. The polar bodies mark the animal pole. Modified from Monroy & Moscona (1979).

rior part of the embryo and eventually gives rise to the musculature of the tail, while the clear transparent cytoplasm becomes the ectoderm. This highly anisotropic structure of the fertilized oocyte prompted embryologists at the turn of the last century to classify such oocytes as mosaic structures.

2. In the sea urchin embryo the organization of the early embryo is quite different (Figure 4.1). After fertilization there is no obvious segregation of cytoplasmic components and although cleavage results in the compartmentalization of the cytoplasm, the blastomeres retain a certain degree of flexibility. Thus, although each blastomere in situ develops into a certain part of the embryo it retains the capacity to differentiate into other tissue types. This capacity can be demonstrated by simple experimentation. If a blastomere is isolated from a two or four cell embryo, it can reorganize itself and give rise to a whole larva. This phenomenon is called regulation. Amphibian and mammalian blastomeres may also be described as regulative. Blastomeres from mosaic embryos do not have this capacity. For example, if the blastomeres of a two cell ascidian embryo are physically separated, each blastomere gives rise to what it would have produced if left in situ, i.e. a half larva. There is a limit to the regulative capacity of sea urchin blastomeres, and a gradient of factors essential for normal development lies along the the A–V axis of the unfertilized sea urchin oocyte. Blastomeres are only capable of regulation if they possess the vegetal factors. As previously mentioned above, the first two cleavages in the sea urchin are longitudinal and therefore all four blastomeres contain some of the vegetal factors. The third cleavage is equatorial, and if the animal blastomeres are separated from the vegetal blastomeres only the latter cells are capable of forming a whole larva. The elegant implantation experiments of Horstadius in the 1920s and 1930s demonstrated that these vegetal factors are in fact distributed in a gradient. Essentially, in the 64-cell stage embryo there are three tiers of vegetal blastomeres: those nearest the animal blastomeres are nominated Veg 1, the next layer Veg 2, and the micromeres

form the distal layer. If an equatorial cut is made through the embryo and the animal half isolated this will only give rise to a permanent blastula. However, if the micromeres from a second embryo are removed and implanted onto this isolated animal half, a normal embryo will develop. A similar though weaker effect is exerted by implanting the Veg 2 blastomeres, but using the Veg 1 blastomeres results in a defective larva.

The process of embryogenesis is complex, involving cell growth, differentiation and movement. In order to coordinate these cellular activities, we expect the embryonic cells to be in communication. This is indeed the case; communicative devices arise early in development and may serve additional roles in the synchronization of early divisions and the determination of the future planes of mitotic spindles. Two types of intercellular junction have been described:

1. Structural junctions such as desmosomes which serve to anchor the cells together.
2. Low resistance junctions such as gap junctions which allow the flow of electrical current and the transfer of small molecules between blastomeres.

The segregation of somatic and germ cell lines in *Ascaris*

The mechanism by which nuclear activity may be irreversibly modified by changes in the cytoplasmic environment has been discussed, and indeed this seems to be the key to understanding the phenomenon of cellular differentiation. Such processes are subtle, and to date they have not been clearly elucidated. In the nematode worm *Ascaris* nuclear differentiation during embryogenesis is more obvious and can be followed by light microscopy. In this worm the somatic cell line segregates from the germ cell line very early during the course of cleavage. During nuclear division the cells of the germ line receive the full chromosome complement, whereas in somatic line cells the tips of the chromosomes are structurally modified and eventually cast off. We may conclude that the somatic cells do not require the full genetic complement for development, whereas the germ cells do require a full complement of genes. During later stages of embryogenesis the somatic cell line differentiates further, forming the various tissues of the adult, but there is no further chromosome elimination.

First stages of development in mammals

In mammals the zygote remains in the oviduct for a few days undergoing cleavage divisions which restore a normal cytoplasmic/nuclear ratio in the cells. The conceptus genome contributes to development from the two cell stage in the

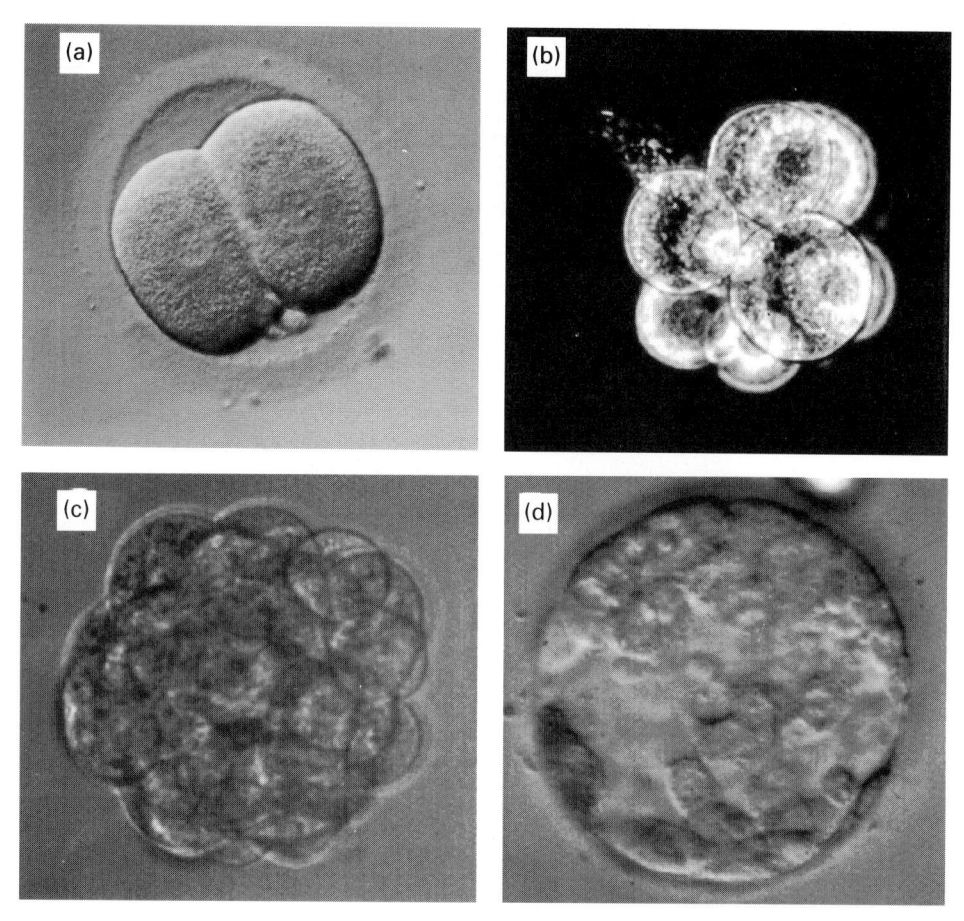

Figure 4.3 The first stages of development in the human: two cells (a), eight cell (b), morula (c), and blastocyst (d). In b and c the zona pellucida has been removed.

mouse and the 4–8 cell stage in the human and large farm animals. At about the third cleavage division the embryo undergoes the process of compaction to form the morula. At this stage there is a significant increase in RNA and protein synthesis and in the synthetic patterns of phospholipids. At the 32 cell stage a second morphological change occurs which gives rise to the blastocyst (Figure 4.3). The form of the blastocyst varies between species, but essentially it is made up of an outer layer of trophectoderm cells and an eccentrically placed inner cell mass layer. The central part of the blastocyst is a fluid filled cavity, the blastocoel. The trophectoderm cells will eventually become the extra-embryonic tissue. This early developmental stage is referred to as the pre-embryo. Throughout these early stages the embryo is enclosed in the zona pellucida, which keeps the cells together during compaction and prevents two

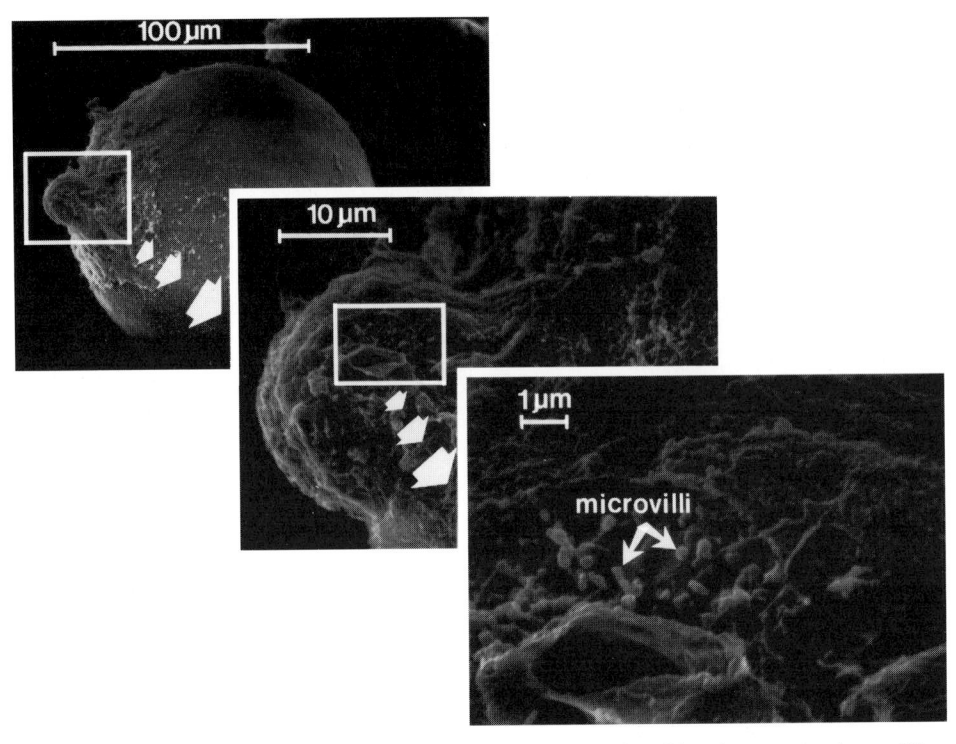

Figure 4.4 Scanning electron micrograph of a hatching human embryo. The microvilli on the surface of the trophectoderm cells are bared owing to internal pressure in the blastocoel and dissolution of the zona pellucida.

embryos fusing and forming a chimera. If the inner cell mass divides at this early stage monozygotic (identical) twins may develop.

During the transition from morula to blastocyst the embryo enters the uterus, where it derives oxygen and metabolic substrates. At the site of implantation the trophectoderm cells produce proteolytic enzymes which digest a passage through the zona pellucida, while in some animals the uterine environment also contains proteolytic enzymes (Figure 4.4). The exposed cell layers make firm physical contact and implantation starts. In the human embryo the first 14–18 days of development are concerned mainly with the differentiation of various extra-embryonic tissues, and only after this time can separate tissues be identified (Figures 4.5 and 4.6).

Further reading

Balinsky, B. (1965) *An Introduction to Embryology.* W. B. Saunders, Philadelphia.
Cole, H. & Cupps, P. (1977) *Reproduction in Domestic Animals.* Academic Press, New York.
Dale, B. (1983) *Fertilization in Animals,* Edward Arnold, London.
Horstadius, S. (1939) The mechanisms of sea urchin development, studied by operative methods. *Biological Reviews.* **14:** 132–179.

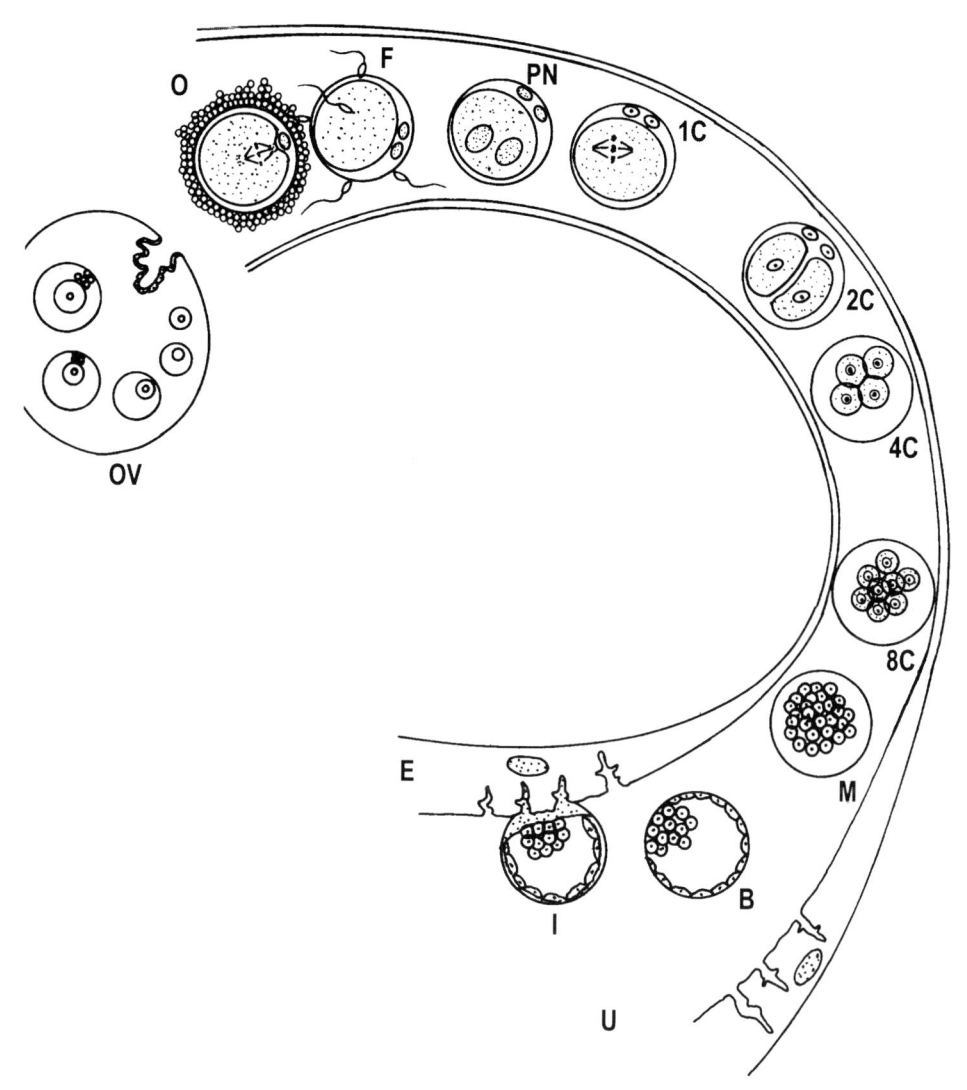

Figure 4.5 Development of the mammalian embryo. The oocytes, released from the ovary (OV), enter the ampulla where they are fertilized (F), and then are transported along the fallopian tube, cleaving to generate the morula stage (M). The blastocyst expands, hatches, and then implants in the endometrium (E) of the uterus (U). From Sathananthan (1993).

Monroy, A. & Moscona, A. (1979) *An Introduction to Developmental Biology*. Chicago University Press.
Sathananthan, H., Ng, S.C., Bongo, A., Trounson, A. & Ratnam, S. (1993) *Visual Atlas of Early Human Development of Assisted Reproductive Technology*. Singapore University Press.

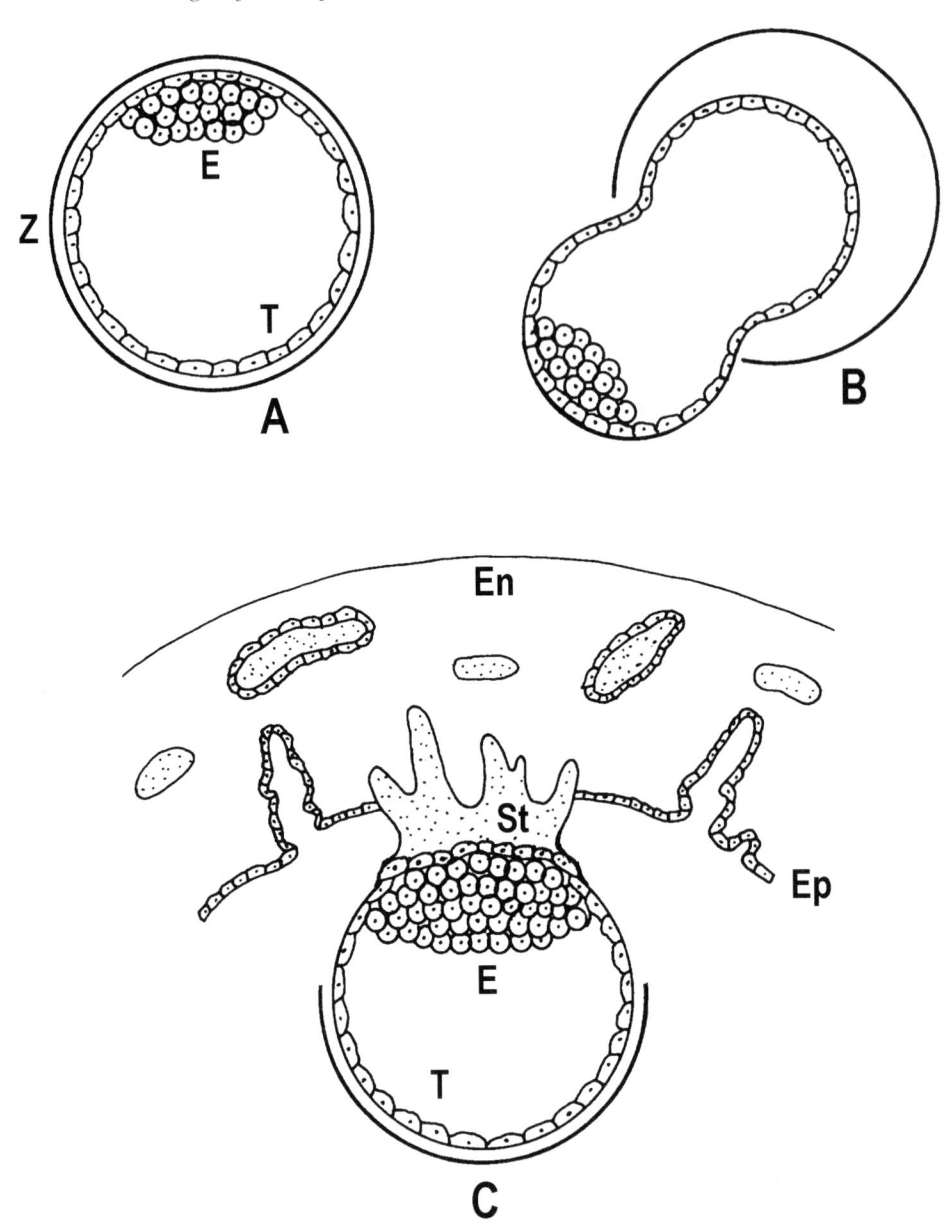

Figure 4.6 Implantation in the mammal. (A) Expanded blastocyst showing the flat layer of trophectoderm cells (T), which will become part of the extra-embryonic tissue and the inner cell mass (E) from which the embryo derives. (B) Shows hatching, probably due in part to the production of a proteolytic-like enzyme by some of the trophectoderm cells. (C) Invasion of the epithelium (Ep) of the endometrium (En).

5

Endocrine control of reproduction

The previous chapters describe gamete biology at the cellular level. Synchrony is essential for correct embryo development, and to understand synchrony a basic knowledge of reproductive endocrinology is fundamental. Although sexual arousal, erection and ejaculation in the male are obviously under cerebral control, it is less obvious that the ovarian and testicular cycles are also coordinated by the brain. For many years after the discovery of the gonadotrophic hormones, follicle stimulating hormone (FSH) and luteinizing hormone (LH), the anterior pituitary gland was considered to be an autonomous organ. Animal experiments in which lesions were induced in the hypothalamus clearly demonstrated the mediation of reproductive processes by the nervous system. The hypothalamus, a small inconspicuous part of the brain lying between the midbrain and the forebrain, controls sexual cycles, growth, pregnancy, lactation, and a wide range of other basic and emotional reactions. Despite its small size the hypothalamus is an extremely complicated structure. Each hypothalamic function is associated with one or more small areas which consist of aggregations of neurons called hypothalamic nuclei. Unlike any other region of the brain, it not only receives sensory inputs from almost every other part of the central nervous system (CNS), but also sends nervous impulses to several endocrine glands and to pathways governing the activity of skeletal muscle, the heart, and smooth muscle. In the context of reproduction, several groups of hypothalamic nuclei are connected to the underlying pituitary gland by neural and vascular connections.

Gonadotrophin hormone releasing hormone (GnRH) is a neurosecretory product of neurons in the hypothalamus which is transported to the anterior pituitary through the portal vessels. GnRH, a decapeptide with the structure (Pyr)-Glu-His-Trp-Ser-Tyr-Gly-Leu-Arg-Pro-Gly-NH_2), is the most important mediator of reproduction by the CNS. Any abnormality in its synthesis, storage, release or action will cause partial or complete failure of gonadal function. GnRH secretion occurs in a pulsatile mode and binds to specific receptors on the plasma membrane of the gonadotroph cells in the pituitary, triggering the inositol triphosphate second messenger system within the cells. This signal induces the movement of secretory granules towards the plasma membrane and eventually the pulsatile secretion of LH and FSH. Continued exposure to GnRH or to a GnRH analogue results in a maintained occupancy of the receptors, uncoupling the receptor from its signal transduction system, and eventually leading to a reduction in LH and FSH secretion (figure 5.1).

In summary, alterations in the output of GnRH, LH and FSH may be achieved by changing the amplitude or frequency of GnRH, or by modulating the response of the gonadotroph cells. In primates, gonadotrophin output is regulated by the ovary. Low circulating levels of oestradiol exert a negative feedback control on LH and FSH secretion, and high maintained levels of oestradiol exert a positive feedback effect. High plasma levels of progesterone enhance the negative feedback effects of oestradiol and hold FSH and LH secretion down to a low level. The secretion of FSH, but not LH, is also regulated by non-steroidal high molecular weight (around 30 000) proteins called inhibins found in follicular fluid: inhibin is found at high levels in late follicular phase plasma of fertile women.

The neuroendocrine mechanisms which regulate testicular function are fundamentally similar to those which regulate ovarian activity. The male hypothalamo–pituitary unit is responsible for the secretion of gonadotrophins which regulate the endocrine and spermatogenic activities of the testis, and this gonadotrophin secretion is subject to feedback regulation. A major difference between male and female reproductive endocrinology is the fact that gamete and steroid hormone production in the male is a continuous process after puberty, and not cyclical as in the female. This is reflected in the absence of positive feedback control of gonadotrophin release by testicular products. In the male, LH stimulates the production of testosterone by the Leydig cells and this testosterone in turn regulates LH secretion by reducing the frequency and amplitude of LH peaks. Although less clearly than in the female, inhibin-like molecules in the male have also been found in testicular extracts, which presumably also regulate FSH secretion. In humans, failure of spermatogenesis is correlated with elevated serum FSH levels, perhaps through reduced inhibin secretion by the testis.

Further reading

Austin, C.R. & Short, R.V. (1972) *Reproduction in Mammals.* Cambridge University Press, Cambridge.

Johnson, M. & Everitt, B. (1990) *Essential Reproduction.* Blackwell Publications, Oxford.

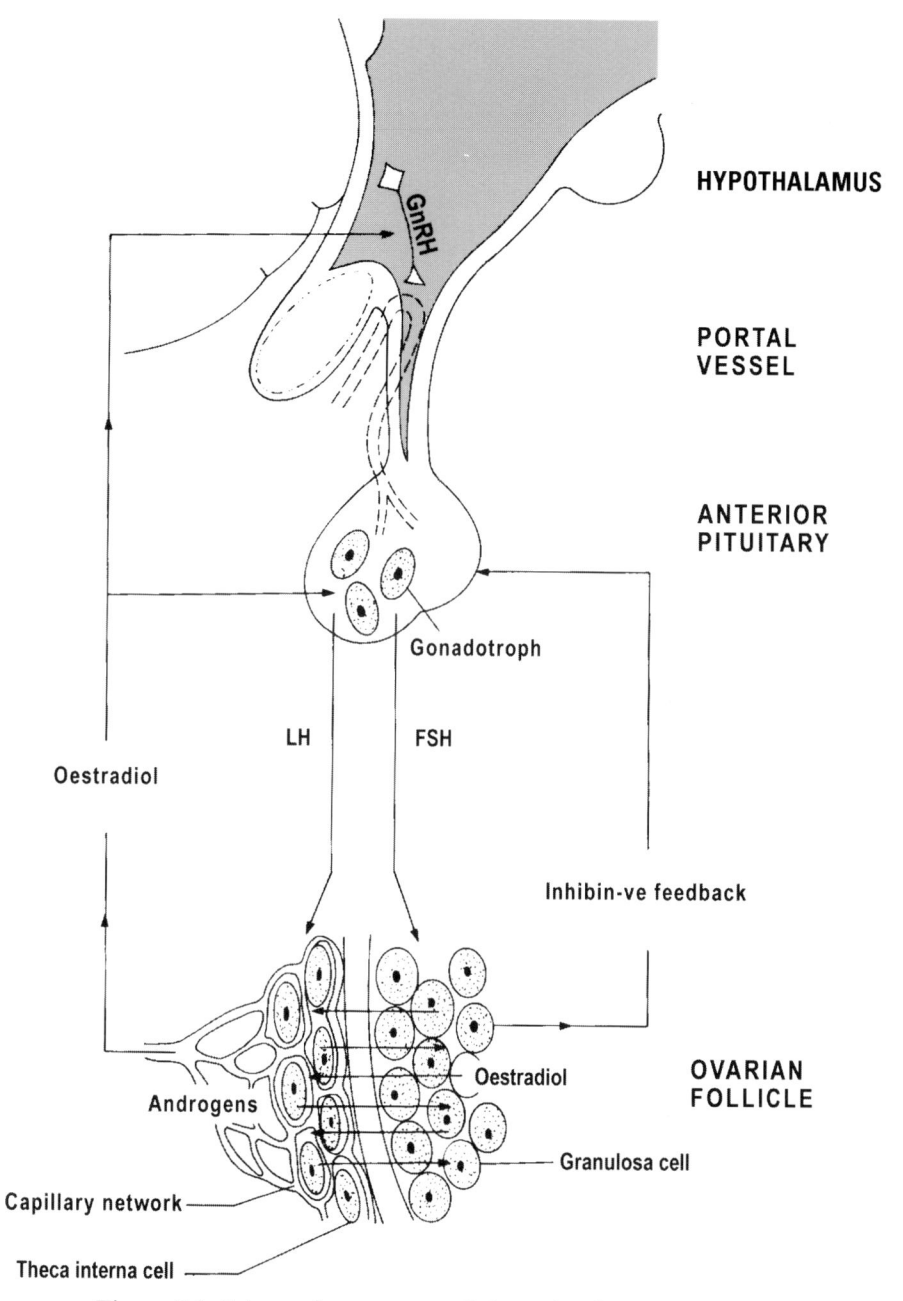

Figure 5.1 Schematic summary of the endocrine control of reproduction in mammals. From Johnson & Everitt (1990).

6
Assisted reproductive technology (ART) in farm animals

Artificial insemination (AI) is the predominant method currently used to increase reproductive potential in agriculture. Although practised in many species, this technique is particularly useful in cattle, where the cost-benefit over natural mating is substantial. In many western countries currently up to 99% of cattle are inseminated artificially. The most common method of semen collection involves the use of an artificial vagina which is designed to simulate natural conditions. This consists of a rigid cylindrical case with a rubber liner, which is lubricated on the inner surface. The space between liner and case is filled with warm water, usually at 40–45 °C, and pressure adjustments may be made by inflating with air. When the male mounts a dummy female the penis is deflected by the operator into the artificial vagina and the ejaculate is collected in a suitably heated receptacle. An alternative method, for use with difficult or young males being taught to mount dummies, is electro-ejaculation using a rectal probe.

There are significant species differences in the volume of semen and the total number of spermatozoa in an ejaculate. The boar, owing to its large testis and to the short duration of its spermatogenic cycle, produces up to 200 ml of semen containing 300×10^6/ml of spermatozoa to give a total of 60×10^9/ml. The bull, in contrast, produces up to 8 ml of semen with a concentration of up to 2000×10^6/ml, to give a final number of 15×10^9/ml. The number of spermatozoa that can be exploited from an animal varies greatly and depends on the frequency of semen collection. A mature dairy bull produces about $13\,000 \times 10^6$ spermatozoa per day. In cattle the cervix is held via the rectum so that a pipette can be guided into the uterus to deposit the semen. Normally 1 ml of semen is deposited, with an optimum number of 10 million spermatozoa. In sheep, due to the folding of the cervix, the spermatozoa are deposited within the first fold of the cervix by means of a fine catheter. In this case more spermatozoa are generally required, and 100 million sperm are usually deposited. The pig, however, requires 2000 million spermatozoa diluted to 50–100 ml, delivered via a corkscrew-shaped catheter similar to the shape of the glans penis of the male.

In humans, washed spermatozoa may be deposited in the uterus using a simple straight catheter to deliver one million to ten million spermatozoa near the fundus, in a small volume of culture medium.

As the fertile life span of spermatozoa in the female tract is limited, as is the ovulation period, the timing of insemination is one of the most important factors in AI. The luteinizing hormone (LH) surge controls the induction of ovulation, and oocyte release occurs 36–40 hours after this surge in the cow and human, 24 hours later in the sheep, and 40–42 hours later in the pig. The optimum time for insemination is 10–12 hours before ovulation. Delayed insemination, which may result in the fertilization of aged oocytes, may lead to polyspermy and anomalous development. Accurate diagnosis of oestrous in farm animals is therefore essential for success in AI. The greatest advantages from AI are as a result of developments in semen storage. Storage medium usually contains a cryoprotectant such as egg yolk, glycerol or dimethyl sulphoxide (DMSO), and the semen sample diluted with cryoprotectant is stored at $-196\ °C$ in liquid nitrogen. Not all semen samples freeze-thaw adequately. Cattle and human spermatozoa are easy to freeze-thaw, while ram spermatozoa present more difficulties and boar sperm is very difficult.

The oestrous cycle in cattle and pigs is 21 days, while in sheep it is 16 days. In any group of animals, the cycles are randomly distributed. Thus pharmacological control of oestrous and ovulation would help to improve the efficiency of AI. Although ovulation may be induced at any stage of the oestrous cycle by gonadotrophins, fertility of the oocyte is impaired if there are high circulating levels of progesterone. Thus gonadotrophic hormones may only be used during the follicular phase of the cycle. In cattle the active corpus luteum that produces progesterone may be squeezed from the ovary by rectal palpation, after which the animal returns to oestrus within a few days. The only promising technique for oestrous synchronization is the use of pituitary inhibitors to suppress natural cycles, followed by releasing the suppression so that all the animals are synchronized. Today gonadotrophin releasing hormone (GnRH) analogues such as buserelin or nafarelin are used to accurately control oestrous in the human. Treatment with exogenous gonadotrophins to induce ovulation is common practice in farm animals and humans alike. This is known as superovulation and leads to an increased number of ovulated follicles. In all species, however, the limiting factor for productivity is the ability of the uterus to support supernumerary embryos. In many species excess foetuses will die in the latter stages of gestation.

Whereas artificial insemination on the farm is a relatively easy technique for improving and managing livestock for the smaller and medium size breeders, larger scale breeders are moving to in vitro methods to increase embryo production and stock management. The long-term objective is to achieve industrial scale production of sex-determined embryos of appropriate genetic merit. These disease-free embryos can then be cryopreserved for later surgical transfer on the farm. Future improvements may be achieved by surgically producing twins and possibly by large-scale cloning, enabling mass embryo transfer to perhaps become normal commercial farm practice.

Cattle ovaries contain thousands of potential oocytes, but the harvesting of these as unfertilized oocytes or embryos by orthodox in vitro fertilization (IVF) technology is usually too costly for serious extensive application of the technique. The large-scale production of cattle embryos by entirely in vitro procedures should be regarded as only the first step towards successful established application of this new technology in commercial practice. On-farm operations need to be simplified to the point where it is possible to thaw IVF embryos and carry out non-surgical transfers in much the same way as applying artificial insemination. When it becomes possible to pre-determine the sex of embryos cheaply and effectively, the provision of bull calves for beef production would have obvious advantages.

Very few of the oocytes present in the ovary are ovulated and made available for fertilization during the reproductive lifespan of the cow. Some reports estimate that as many as 150 000 primary follicles are present in the ovary of the calf at birth. Although current super-ovulation techniques can increase the reproductive capacity of the cow substantially, such measures only utilize a small proportion of the total number of oocytes in the ovary. Ovaries from slaughtered cows offer a valid alternative. Aspiration of follicular oocytes, using either a pipette or syringe and needle, is the most common method of recovering immature cattle oocytes for large-scale embryo production. The interval between slaughter and the start of recovery operations is important in recovering oocytes from slaughterhouse ovaries. Cattle ovaries may be stored at a temperature of about 25 °C for at least 11 hours without compromising oocyte fertilization and normal embryo development. Within the intact bovine vesicular follicle, the oocyte and the surrounding mass of cumulus cells form a structural and functional syncytium. The cumulus oophorus also acts as a bridge between the cells of the stratum granulosum and the oocyte, allowing molecules to be transferred from the granulosa cells to the oocyte.

The current maturation process for cattle oocytes involves adding five million cumulus/granulosa cells to each 1 ml of medium, with 20 or more oocytes per 2 ml volume. The culture media used for in vitro maturation ranges from simple physiological solutions to complex types containing amino acids, vitamins, purines and other compounds designed for general cell culture. A flux culture system is routinely employed, with gentle agitation of the dishes in which oocytes are matured. Temperature is maintained at 39 °C, the core temperature of the cow. For successful cattle IVF, it is essential to have a reliable means of artificially capacitating sperm. The first effective capacitating procedure employed in cattle IVF was that of Brackett, who used a high ionic strength (HIS) medium, but the use of heparin is more common. This glycosaminoglycan is present in the reproductive tract of the cow and is believed to be involved in the natural process of capacitation in the live animal. In vitro fertilization of artificially matured oocytes is carried out in microdroplets of 50 μL of medium at pH 7.8, with an estimated one million spermatozoa per ml. There is considerable variation between different bulls in the fertilizing capacity of their semen, not only in terms of fertilization rates but also in the subsequent yield of embryos. Semen for cattle IVF should be obtained from bulls with a proven record of high fertility. The oocyte remains surrounded by layers of expanded cumulus cells after maturation. In the cow, these cells are rapidly eroded once the oocyte moves into the oviduct. In an effort to make oocytes more accessible to sperm, some of these cell layers can be removed, either by mechanical stripping in a pipette or with hyaluronidase treatment. As with maturation, the efficiency of the fertilization process can be markedly influenced by temperature. Spermatozoal penetration in bovine oocytes is less than 1% at 37 °C, but increases to 90% at 39 °C, the core temperature of the cow.

Research is still needed to accummulate reliable data on pregnancy and calving rates with in vitro embryos, compared with the figures already available from the use of in vivo cultured embryos or those obtained from superovulated donor cattle after conventional embryo transfer recovery. There is some evidence to suggest that the in vitro cultured embryos contain a smaller number of inner cell mass (ICM) cells.

Microsurgery was first used to study live mammalian oocytes in the late 1940s, and the 1950s and 1960s saw an increased interest in mammalian experimental embryology. A major influence during this period was T. P. Lin, who performed numerous studies on the technical and experimental nature of oocyte microsurgery. Lin and co-workers also studied the effect of partial microsuction of the egg cytoplasm on the development and transplantation of chromosomes into mammalian oocytes. Microsurgical approaches to the study of early mammalian development progressed with the use of exogenous gonadotrophins to increase the number of oocytes ovulated and consequently the number of pre-implantation embryos available for experimental manipulation. A fundamental observation was made in 1968, when a single blastomere taken from an eight cell rabbit embryo gave rise to a live birth.

During the past 30 years a fascinating array of manipulations have been carried out on the pre-implantation animal embryo. The majority of these experiments have involved the addition or removal of cells, or the transplantation of nuclei. More recently, exogenous DNA has been introduced into the zygote or early embryo to study the function of gene products, the regulation of gene expression and the generation of transgenic animals. Various microsurgical experiments have been devised to study the fate of early differentiating tissues, the contribution of cells from the ICM and the trophectoderm, and the timing of X-chromosome inactivation. In 1961, Andresz Tarkowski first produced a chimera, and in 1968 Richard Gardner generated chimeras by injecting cells into a blastocyst. In addition to intraspecific chimeras, a number of scientists have used interspecific chimeras to study early embryogenesis. This technique enables an embryo from one species to develop within the placenta and uterus of a second species, with subsequent delivery of viable chimeras; this has been achieved using the sheep and the goat.

Another microsurgical approach involves the removal of blastomeres in order to study the fate of partial embryos. In the 1980s, blastomere separation was utilized to produce genetically identical twins, triplets and quadruplets. These techniques have obvious implications in agriculture, where successful sexing of embryos and the production of two or more embryos from one embryo are of enormous cost-benefit to the farmer. Early attempts to transplant whole nuclei in mammalian zygotes to produce clones for animal husbandry have been disappointing. On the other hand, the production of transgenic animals by direct microinjection of DNA into one of the zygote pronuclei has been relatively successful. Approximately 100 linear DNA molecules in a volume of one picolitre are injected into the pronucleus. The DNA is integrated into the recipient DNA during the early cleavage stages and the genetic trait is transmitted to the offspring.

The term transgene describes novel DNA sequences introduced following laboratory manipulation of the zygote. The majority of transgenic animals have been made by pronuclear injection of naked linear DNA. A great deal of excitement accompanied a report that foreign DNA mixed with mouse spermatozoa prior to in vitro fertilization, resulted in approximately 30% of pups carrying integrated transgenes. Unfortunately, a concerted international effort to repeat these results has been unsuccessful. The current gene transfer method of choice remains pronuclear injection. Fertilized oocytes are recovered from superovulated donors at the pronuclear stage (i.e. prior to formation of a single diploid nucleus). The injection procedure requires two micromanipulators to support the holding and injection pipettes respectively, and an inverted microscope with Hoffman optics. Embryos are held on a fire-polished glass holding pipette which is connected to a hydraulic control system. A second finely drawn pipette is introduced into the male pronucleus and several hundred copies of the gene construct are injected. Injection is accompanied by pronuclear swelling and probable chromosome damage (mechanical damage may actually be necessary for transgene integration). Injected embryos are incubated briefly to assess survival and then returned to the ampullae of synchronized females. There are developmental and physiological differences between species which reduce the efficiency of gene transfer in farm animals. While mouse pronuclei are readily visible with differential interference contrast (DIC), ungulate embryos contain a large number of lipid granules which tend to obscure internal structure. The pronuclei in the sheep can be seen under DIC in up to 90% of embryos, but in pigs and cattle, centrifugation is required to sequester these granules to one end of the zygote. The efficiency of gene transfer in farm animals is further reduced because small numbers of embryos are obtained per female.

The main disadvantages of pronuclear injection are effects due to the unpredictability of the site of incorporation, and poor reproducibility of experiments due to random incorporation. In addition we can only add, and not remove sequences. The embryonic stem (ES) cell system is now well documented as an alternative route into the germline of mice which can potentially overcome all of these problems. An additional bonus is the possibility, through ES cells, for the application of site-directed mutagenesis to animals. The ES cell system capitalizes on the capacity of a subpopulation of embryonic cells to proliferate in the undifferentiated state in culture, while maintaining their ability to differentiate fully in vivo (totipotency). When reintroduced into the blastocoele cavity of early embryos, ES cells frequently contribute to the germ line. Hence, pigmented ES cells in albino embryos give rise to chimeric animals whose tissues (including gonads), are a mosaic of host embryo (albino) and ES (pigmented) genotypes. If chimeras are mated to albino females a proportion and, in some cases, all of the offspring will be pigmented, demonstrating the germline transmission of ES-derived DNA.

New technologies such as in vitro maturation, in vitro fertilization, improved culture systems, embryo biopsy and nuclear transfer will dramatically increase the efficiency with which transgenics can be produced. In farm animals, most of the effort has been directed towards the introduction of extra copies of growth hormone genes. At the phenotypic level, results have been disappointing and appropriate genes for the improvement of quantitative traits still need to be identified. Engineering of the mammary gland as a source of recombinant protein is promising, although levels of recombinant protein secretion are constrained by our limited understanding of gene expression.

Nuclear transplantation of embryos has brought to the realm of researchers and animal breeders the possibility of producing large quantities of genetically identical animals by cloning. The technology of cloning started in amphibian embryos in the 1950s. Frog eggs were activated by pricking with a glass needle which causes rotation, bringing the animal pole to lie uppermost. The chromosomes are visualized as a black dot that can be extirpated surgically, or can be effectively ablated with laser or ultraviolet irradiation. A proportion of the embryos derived from the transplantation of nuclei from undetermined embryonic cells (blastula and gastrula stage) were able to support development into normal adults indicating that at least some of these cells are totipotent. Studies carried out using nuclei from determined regions of larvae have shown that only around 0.2% will develop to adults and another 4% will arrest at the larval stage (pluripotent nuclei).

As the volume of the mammalian oocyte is one thousand times smaller than that of frog oocytes it is not surprising that more refined methods of microsurgery were required before the development of techniques for nuclear transplantation could be usefully applied to mammals. The successful microinjection of embryonic nuclei into the cytoplasm of rabbit and mouse zygotes suggested that nuclei from later embryonic stages were able to participate with the oocyte genome in supporting pre-implantation development. The first report of mice born from nuclear transplantation came from the work of Illmensee and Hoppe in 1981, showing that nuclei derived from the inner cell mass rather than the trophectoderm of mouse blastocysts were able to support development to the morula-blastocyst stage in 34% of the transferred embryos and that 19% of these would develop to term. These reports brought many scientists to speculate that this technique would provide a means of making an infinite number of genetically identical copies from a single embryo. In 1983 McGrath and Solter fused nuclei in a membrane-bound karyoplast to enucleated pronuclear zygotes. Fusion is performed by injecting a small amount of a solution of inactivated Sendai virus which causes the membranes of the karyoplast and the enucleated embryo to fuse within a few minutes of manipulation. Contrary to the poor levels of success obtained using Illmensee and Hoppe's invasive technique, this method proved to be virtually 100% successful.

By using this non-invasive technique, several laboratories have shown that nuclei derived from mouse two-cell blastomeres are only able to support in vitro development to morula-blastocyst stages. Steen Willadsen in 1986 first reported the development to blastocyst and to term of sheep embryos derived from the transplantation of eight-cell blastomere nuclei to enucleated oocytes. The relevance of these findings was not exclusively related to the ability of a single eight-cell blastomere to support development, as this had already been shown in chimeric studies. The significant feature of this observation was that the resulting fused embryo would develop and differentiate as if commencing from the time of fertilization. This indicates that the oocyte cytoplasm has the capacity to reprogramme the developmental pathway of the donor nucleus. The optimal stage for utilizing oocytes after ovulation has not yet been determined, but a short period of aging seems to increase the potential for development. In general, secondary oocytes are obtained directly from the oviduct either during surgical intervention or at slaughter.

One limitation for the use of oocytes as recipient cytoplasm concerns the enucleation procedure. With the exception of the rabbit, metaphase chromosomes cannot be readily visualized in secondary oocytes from farm species due to the presence of large lipid vesicles in the cytoplasm. Consequently, the position of the first polar body is used to indicate the position of the chromosomal plate for aspiration of the chromosomes and surrounding cytoplasm. Non-invasive methods for nuclear transplantation rely on an effective method for fusing the nuclear (karyoplast) and cytoplasmic (cytoplast) portions of two different cells.

Several methods are available for fusion, some of which are either unreliable and toxic, such as polyethylene glycol and lysolecithin, or laborious and dangerous, such as inactivated Sendai virus. Electrofusion has been successfully used to fuse blastomeres and for nuclear transplantation experiments in mammalian embryos derived from species as diverse as mice, rabbit, sheep, cattle and pigs. Fusion seems to be a result of the reversible instability of the plasma membranes in the zone of membrane contact between the cytoplasm and nuclear donor cells. Successful fusion can be attained using a large range of parameters for the direct current fusing pulse. Values of around 1 kV/cm field intensity with durations of 50–100 microseconds are commonly used. Alternating current pulses may be used to align the cells so that their membranes are positioned perpendicular to the electrical field where conditions for fusion are most appropriate. The preceding AC pulse is particularly important when fusing enucleated oocytes to cells with reduced diameters since the polarization caused by the AC field will help to bring their membranes into contact for the DC fusing pulse. Experiments with mouse pronuclear zygotes have indicated that cell cycle stage synchrony between nucleus and cytoplasm is beneficial for further development in vitro. This observation has been further extended to transplantations between two-cell embryos where asynchronous exchanges were highly deleterious to further development. This effect may be explained either by the disruption of the cell cycle oscillatory mechanisms or by incompatible nucleo–cytoplasmic interactions in controlling critical developmental steps. It is important to note some of the possible disadvantages in the cloning procedure. One aspect concerns the decrease in genetic variability caused by inbreeding. Large foundation populations should be obtained when using cloning in conjuction with multiple ovulation and embryo transfer selection schemes. It is also important to verify the degree to which cytoplasmic inheritance can influence animal production as clones will not only be exposed to different uterine and neonatal environments, but also to a different ooplasm. The possible maternal inheritance of mitochondrial and centriole genomes are examples of differences that may arise between clones derived by nuclear transplantation. Another potential factor for consideration of genetic variation is the random inactivation of x chromosomes in females.

Further reading

Cole, H. & Cupps, P. (1977) *Reproduction in Domestic Animals.* Academic Press, New York.
Gordon, I. & Lu, K. (1990) Production of embryos in vitro and its impact on livestock production. *Theriogenology* **33:** 77–87.
Hafez, E. (1987) *Reproduction in Farm Animals.* Lea and Febiger, New York.
King, T. (1966) Nuclear transplantation in amphibia. *Methods in Cell Biology* **2:** 1.
McLaren, A. (1984) Methods and success of nuclear transplantation in mammals. *Nature* **309:** 671–672
Palmiter, R. & Brinster, R. (1986) Germline transformation of mice. *Annual Reviews in Genetics* **20:** 465–499.

7

Micromanipulation, assisted reproductive technology, and the future

Micromanipulation of cells dates from the turn of the last century when biologists and physiologists used a variety of manipulator systems to dissect or record from cells. Experiments in which sperm were injected into eggs around the mid-1960s were primarily designed to investigate the early events of fertilization, i.e. the role of membrane fusion, activation of the oocyte, and the formation of the pronuclei. Two series of early experiments by independent groups demonstrated major species differences. Hiramoto showed in the 1960s that microinjection of spermatozoa into unfertilised sea urchin oocytes did not induce activation of the oocyte or condensation of the sperm nucleus, whereas others demonstrated the opposite in frog oocytes. Ryuzo Yanagimachi and his group later demonstrated that isolated hamster nuclei could develop into pronuclei after microinjection into homologous eggs, and a similar result was obtained when freeze-dried human spermatozoa were injected into a hamster egg. These experiments indicated that during activation of mammalian oocytes, membrane fusion events may be bypassed without compromising the initiation of development. The experiments not only provided information on the mechanism of fertilization, but led to a new technique in clinical embryology.

The first clinical application of microinsemination techniques was partial zona dissection (PZD) developed by Jacques Cohen and colleagues to aid fertilization in human oocytes (Figure 7.1). This mechanical technique involves breaching a slit in the zona pellucida with a sharp glass micropipette and subsequently placing the dissected oocyte into a suspension of spermatozoa, on the assumption that sperm entry is facilitated by the slit. In the same year, S.C. Ng and colleagues in Singapore reported the first pregnancy from subzonal sperm injection (SUZI), where several spermatozoa are inserted into the perivitelline space (Figure 7.2). In 1990 the same group reported activation of human oocytes following intracytoplasmic injection of human spermatozoa, and in

68 *Micromanipulation and the future*

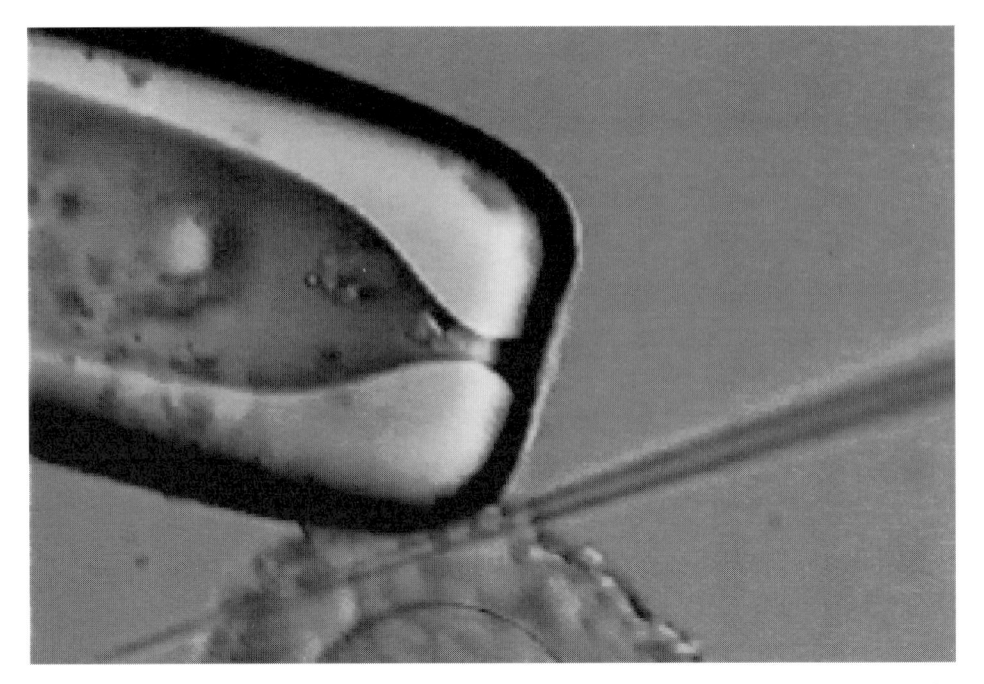

Figure 7.1 The last stages of partial zona drilling where friction between the inserted needle and the holding pipette results in a slit in the zona pellucida.

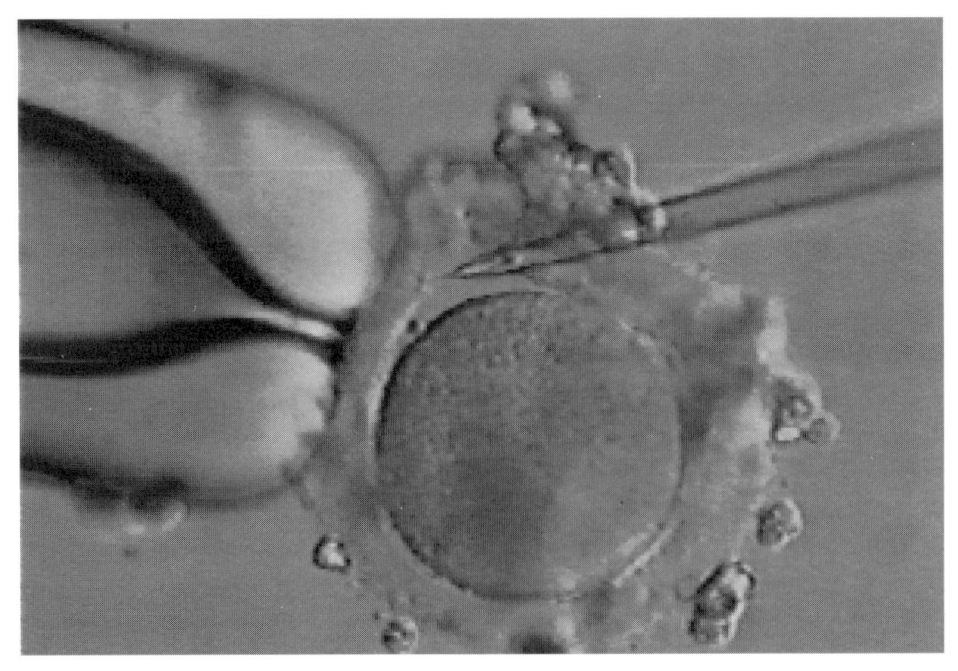

Figure 7.2 Injection of a spermatozoon into the perivitelline space of a human oocyte (SUZI).

SZI   **ICSI**

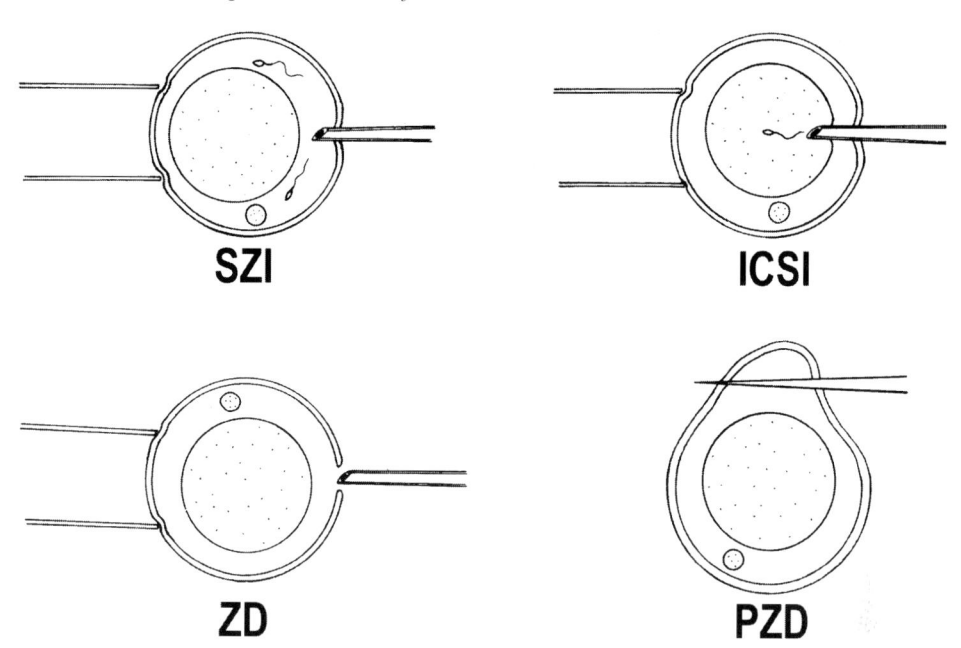

ZD   **PZD**

Figure 7.3 Microinsemination techniques include subzonal injection (SZI), intracytoplastic sperm injection (ICSI), zona drilling (ZD), and partial zona dissection (PZD).

1992 Palermo and VanSterteigheim in Brussels reported the first pregnancies from this technique of intracytoplasmic sperm injection (ICSI). Since the time of these pioneering reports more than 2000 ICSI babies have been born worldwide (Figure 7.3).

A second micromanipulation technique that has proved to be useful in improving the outcome of assisted reproductive technology (ART) in humans was developed by Jacques Cohen and colleagues in 1990. They demonstrated that assisted hatching (AH), cutting a slit in the zona pellucida or dissolving a hole in the zona with an acid solution, facilitated implantation of the human embryo in selected cases (see Chapter 12).

Using micromanipulation techniques for embryo biopsy, the early 1990s have seen the development of pre-implantation genetic diagnosis as an alternative to traditional prenatal diagnosis and recurrent abortions for couples who are at risk of transmitting an inherited disease to their children. Couples at risk of bearing children with sex-linked diseases which affect male offspring, such as haemophilia and muscular dystrophy, may be helped by pre-determining the sex of the embryo before it implants.

Obviously, the easiest and most cost-effective method would be to sort X- from Y-bearing spermatozoa in the ejaculate. The only established difference between X and Y chromosome-bearing spermatozoa is the quantity of DNA in the sex chromosome. Many physical, chemical and immunological methods for separating X and Y spermatozoa have been proposed, but as yet there is no conclusive technique to date for separating human sperm. In 1973 it was suggested that human Y spermatozoa are enriched when swimmimg downwards in albumin columns; since that time over 100 papers have been published, with both positive and negative reports as to its success in influencing the sex ratio. The only scientifically proven method of separating X- and Y-bearing vital mammalian spermatozoa is the use of a flow cytometry sorter. Spermatozoa are labelled with a fluorescent DNA dye (Bisbenzimide) and exposed to ultraviolet excitation. Spermatozoa are deflected into one or other direction depending on the intensity of the signal, and X- and Y-bearing sperm separately collected. Unfortunately the technique is slow, allowing only 300 000 spermatozoa to be processed per hour, and therefore it is not suitable for artificial insemination. In addition, it is highly likely that the DNA fluorochrome is teratogenetic, and, finally, the modified cell sorter is extremely expensive. To date, the only successful method for sexing pre-implantation embryos is by embryo biopsy. The couple undergo traditional in vitro fertilization (IVF) treatment to generate embryos, and at the 6–10 cell stage, two cells from each embryo are biopsied, using a blunt micropipette (Figure 7.4). The cells are analysed either by fluorescent in situ hybridization (FISH) or by the polymerase chain reaction (PCR) to determine the sex of each embryo. These procedures may be carried out in 4–6 hours, and embryos judged to be disease-free may then be transferred to the patient. The same technique using PCR has also been successfully developed to screen embryos for diseases carried by autosomal chromosomes such as cystic fibrosis and certain forms of anaemia. FISH can also be used to investigate embryos from couples who repeatedly produce abnormally developing IVF embryos. In the clinical setting, pre-implantation diagnosis is a highly specialized and labor-intensive technology which requires not only a highly competent IVF team of exceptionally high standards and micromanipulation facilities, but also a molecular biology laboratory and team able to carry out the FISH and PCR techniques. Input from geneticists is also required for selection and counselling of patients, as well as analysis of the embryos before transfer. To date there are 15 clinics worldwide who are able to offer this treatment to patients, and at the beginning of 1996, 34 babies had been born, all of whom are developing normally.

In Chapter 6 we described technologies which have been applied to large agricultural animals, such as cloning, nuclear transfer and the use of stem cells, etc. This area of research has contributed vastly to our understanding of cell biology

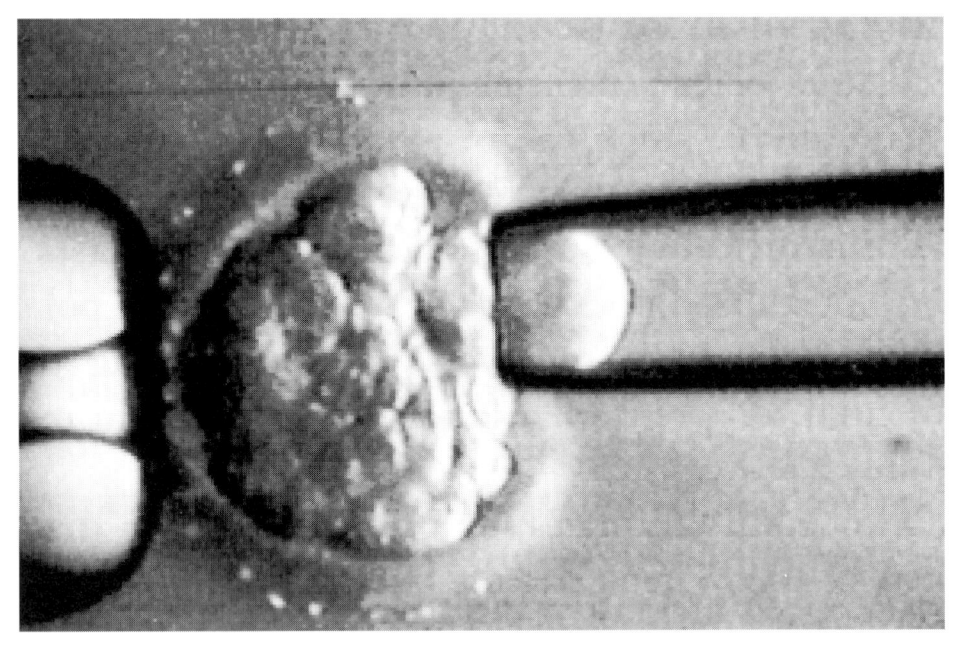

Figure 7.4 Removal of a blastomere from a human embryo for preimplantation diagnosis. By courtesy of Alan Handyside, London.

and the mechanisms involved in reproductive biology and normal embryo development. There have also been significant contributions in the field of cell cycle control, which contribute to our knowledge of diseases caused by uncontrolled cell division, such as cancer.

Obviously, human clinical embryology is an area where many of these technologies may not be applied, and legislation in most countries forbids these types of embryo manipulation in a clinical environment. Due to the inefficiency of human IVF and to the fact that its aim is to achieve the birth of a healthy baby for as many couples as possible, opportunities for clinical reseach on the early embryo are very limited, and restricted to material donated for research with the full knowledge and consent of the donating couple. There are large differences between species, so our ultimate goal of improving clinical treatment by improving the efficiency of IVF will only be reached by understanding human fertilization and implantation. This will only emerge from studies on human gametes and embryos, and clinical scientists working in reproductive medicine must use every opportunity to maximise opportunties for observation and research in order to add to our knowledge in a responsible and effective manner. We hope that authorities influencing future legislation will not ignore this need for basic research, so fundamental for any other branch of medical science.

Further reading

Cohen, J. (1991) Assisted hatching of human embryos. *Journal of In Vitro Fertilization and Embryo Transfer* **8:** 179-189.

Cohen, J., Alikani, M., Trowbridge, J. & Rosenwaks, Z. (1992) Implantation enhancement by selective assisted hatching using zona drillling of embryos with poor prognosis. *Human Reproduction* **7:** 685–691.

Grifo, J. A., Boyle, A. & Fischer, E. (1990) Pre-embryo biopsy and analysis of blastomeres by in situ hybridisation. *American Journal of Obstetrics and Gynaecology* **163:** 2013–2019.

Handyside, A.H., Kontogianni, E.H., Hardy, K., & Winston, R.M.L. (1990) Pregnancies from biopsied human preimplantation embryos sexed by Y-specific DNA amplification. *Nature* **344:** 768–770.

Handyside, A. (1991) Pre-implantation diagnosis by DNA amplification. In: (Chapman, M., Grudzinskas, G., Chard, T., & Maxwell, A. eds), *The embryo*, Springer Verlag, Amsterdam.

Harper, J.C. & Handyside, A.H. (1994) The current status of preimplantation diagnosis. *Current Obstetrics and Gynaecology* **4:** 143–149.

Harper, J.C., Coonan, E. & Ramaekers, F.C.S. (1994) Identification of the sex of human preimplantation embryos in two hours using an improved spreading method and fluorescent in-situ hybridization (FISH) using directly labelled probes. *Human Reproduction* **9:** 721–724.

Munné, S., Alikani, M., Levron, J., Tomkin, G., Palermo, G., Grifo, J. & Cohen, J. (1995) Fluorescent in situ hybridisation in human blastomeres. In: (Hedon, B., Bringer, J., & Mares, P. eds), *Fertility and Sterility.* IFFS-95, The Parthenon Publishing Group, pp. 425–438.

8
The clinical in vitro fertilization laboratory

Introduction

In the armoury of medical technology that now exists for the alleviation of disease and improvement in the quality of life, there is nothing to match the unique contribution of assisted reproductive technology. There is no other life experience that matches the birth of a baby in significance and importance. The responsibility of nurturing and watching children grow and develop alters the

---

The Assisted Conception Treatment Cycle

- Consultation: history, examination, investigation, counselling
- Pituitary downregulation with GnRH agonist
- Baseline assessment
- Gonadotrophin stimulation
- Follicular phase monitoring
    - ultrasound+endocrinology
- HCG administration to induce ovulation
- Oocyte retrieval (OCR)
- In vitro fertilization
- Embryo transfer
- Supernumerary embryo cryopreservation
- Luteal phase support
- Day 15 pregnancy text
- Follow-up pregnancy tests: day 20, 25, 30
- Day 35 ultrasound assessment

appreciation of life and health, with a resulting long-term impact upon individuals, families, and, ultimately, society. Thus, the combination of oocyte and sperm to create an embryo with the potential to develop into a unique individual cannot be regarded lightly, as merely another form of invasive medical technology, but must be treated with the respect and responsibility due to the most fundamental areas of human life.

Successful assisted reproduction involves the careful coordination of both a medical and a scientific approach to each couple who undertake a treatment cycle, with close collaboration between doctors, scientists, nurses, and counsellors. Only meticulous attention to detail at every step of each patient's treatment can optimize their chance of delivering a healthy baby. Appropriate patient selection, ovarian stimulation, monitoring, and timing of oocyte retrieval should provide the in vitro fertilization (IVF) laboratory with viable gametes capable of producing healthy embryos. It is the responsibility of the IVF laboratory to ensure a stable, non-toxic, pathogen-free environment with optimum parameters for oocyte fertilization and embryo development. The first part of this book reveals the complexity of variables involved in assuring successful fertilization and embryo development in animal systems, together with the fascinating and elegant systems of control which have been elucidated at the molecular level. It goes without saying that human in vitro fertilization must of necessity involve systems of at least equal, if not greater, complexity, and it is essential for the clinical biologist to be aware that control mechanisms exist which are exquisitely sensitive to even apparently minor changes in the environment of gametes and embryos, in particular, temperature, pH, and any other factors which potentially affect cells at the molecular level. Multiple variables are involved, so the basic science of each step must be carefully controlled, while allowing for individual variation between patients and between treatment cycles. In addition, in this current era of rapidly evolving technology, the success of new innovations in technique and technology can only be gauged by comparison with a standard of efficient and reproducible established procedures. The IVF laboratory therefore has a duty and responsibility not only to ensure that a strict discipline of cleanliness and sterile technique is adhered to throughout all procedures, but also to produce and maintain daily records, with systematic data analysis and reports.

Setting up a laboratory: equipment and facilities

The design of an IVF laboratory should provide a distraction- and accident-free environment in which concentrated attention can be comfortably and safely dedicated to each manipulation, with sensible and logical planning of work stations which are practical and easy to clean. Priority must be given to minimizing the potential for introducing infection or contamination from any source, and therefore the tissue culture area should allow for the highest standards of sterile technique, with all floors, surfaces and components easy to clean on a daily basis. Ideally, the space should be designated as a restricted access area, with facilities for changing into clean operating theatre dress and shoes before entry.

Careful consideration should be given to the physical manoeuvres involved, ensuring ease and safety of movement between areas, in order to minimize the possibility of accidents. Bench height, adjustable chairs, microscope eye height, and efficient use of space and surfaces all contribute to a working environment that minimizes distraction and fatigue. The location of storage areas and equipment such as incubators and centrifuges should be logically planned for efficiency and safety within each working area; the use of mobile laboratory components allows flexibility to meet changing requirements.

Basic essential equipment required for routine IVF includes:

1. Dissecting, inverted, and light microscopes
2. Incubator with accurately regulated temperature and CO_2
3. Centrifuge for sperm preparation
4. Warmed stages or surfaces for culture manipulations
5. Refrigerator/freezer
6. Dry heat oven for drying and sterilizing

A video camera system is also recommended for teaching, assessment, and records (patients receive enormous satisfaction and psychological support from observing their oocytes and embryos on a video screen).

When choosing these expensive items of equipment, ensure that not only is each easy to use and maintain, but that servicing and repairs can be quickly and efficiently obtained. Routine schedules of cleaning, maintenance, and servicing must be established for each item of equipment, and checklist records maintained for daily, weekly, monthly, and annual schedules of cleaning and maintenance of all items used, together with checks for restocking and expiry dates of supplies.

Incubators

Two types of gas phase have been successfully used: 5% CO_2 in air, and the triple gas mixture of 5% CO_2, 5% O_2, 90% N_2. An atmosphere of 5% CO_2 is required to maintain correct pH in bicarbonate buffered culture media systems in order to maintain a physiological pH of just under 7.5. This equilibrium is affected by both temperature and atmospheric pressures, and some laboratories use 6.0% CO_2 in their incubators.

Carefully calibrated and accurately controlled CO_2 incubators are critical to successful IVF; the choice of a humidified or non-humidified incubator depends upon the type of tissue culture system used: whereas humidity is required for standard four-well 'open' culture, the use of an equilibrated overlay of mineral oil allows the use of incubators without humidity. Dry incubators in general carry less risk of fungal contamination, and are easier to clean. The incubator must be monitored with twice-daily CO_2 level and temperature readings, in order to quickly detect and correct fluctuations. Also bear in mind that the CO_2 display is not necessarily always correct, and carry out a calibration procedure (e.g. FYRITE) as part of the maintenance routine.

Standard maintenance should also include occasional monitoring of temperature stability, using an independent thermocouple record over a 24 hour period.

The inside walls and doors should be washed with sterile water weekly, and a yearly inspection and general servicing by the supplier is recommended.

Repeated opening and closing of the incubator affects the stability of the tissue culture environment; using a small benchtop mini-incubator during oocyte retrievals and manipulations helps to minimize disturbance of the storage incubator.

Supplies

A basic list of supplies is outlined at the end of this chapter; the exact combination required will depend upon the tissue culture system and techniques of manipulation used. Disposables supplies are used whenever possible and must be guaranteed non-toxic tissue culture grade, in particular the culture vessels, needles, collecting system and catheters for oocyte aspiration and embryo transfer.

Disposable high quality glass pipettes are required for gamete and embryo manipulations; these must be soaked and rinsed with tissue culture grade sterile water and dry heat sterilized before use. In preparing to handle gametes or embryos, examine each pipette and rinse with sterile medium to ensure that it is clean and residue-free.

Daily cleaning routine

During the course of procedures any spillage should be immediately cleaned with dry tissue. No detergent or alcohol should be used whilst oocytes/embryos

Setting up a laboratory: equipment and facilities 77

are being handled. Should it be necessary to use either of the above, allow residual traces to evaporate for a period of at least 20 minutes before removing oocytes/embryos from incubators.

At the end of each day:

1. Heat seal, double bag, and dispose of all waste from procedures
2. Remove all pipette holders for washing and sterilizing before re-use.
3. Re-seal and re-sterilize pipette canisters
4. Clean flow hoods, work benches, and all equipment by washing with a solution of distilled water and 7X laboratory detergent (Flow Laboratories), followed by wiping with 70% methylated spirit.
5. Prepare each work station for the following day's work, with clean rubbish bags, pipette holder, and Pasteur pipettes.

Washing procedures

If the laboratory has a system for preparation of ultrapure water, particular attention must be paid to instructions for maintenance and chemical cleaning. Water purity is essential for washing procedures, and the system should be periodically checked for organic contamination and endotoxins.

Pipettes

1. Soak new pipettes overnight in fresh Analar or Milli-Q water, ensuring that they are completely covered.
2. Drain the pipettes and rinse with fresh water.
3. Drain again and dry at 100 °C for 1–2 hours.
4. Place in a clean pipette canister (tips forward), and dry heat sterilize for 3 hours at 180 °C.
5. After cooling, record date and use within 1 month of sterilization.

Non-disposable items (handle with non-powdered gloves, rinsed in purified water)

1. Soak in distilled water containing 3–5% 7X (Flow Laboratories).
2. Sonicate small items for 5–10 minutes in an ultrasonic cleaning bath.
3. Rinse eight times with distilled water, then twice with Analar or Milli-Q water.
4. Dry, seal in aluminium foil or double wrap in autoclave bags as appropriate.
5. Autoclave, or dry heat sterilize at 180 °C. for 3 hours.
6. Record date of sterilization, and store in a clean, dust free area.

Tissue culture media

A great deal of scientific research and analysis has been applied to the development of media which will successfully support the growth and development of human embryos, and many controlled studies have shown fertilization and cleavage to be satisfactory in a variety of simple and complex media. Edwards & Brody have recently published a comprehensive review. Rigorous quality control is essential in media preparation, including the source of all ingredients, especially the water, which must be endotoxin-free, low in ion content, and guaranteed free of organic molecules and microorganisms. Each batch of culture media prepared must be checked for osmolality (285 ± 2 mOsm/kg) and pH (7.35–7.45), and subjected to quality control procedures with sperm survival or mouse embryo toxicity before use.

Commercially prepared, pre-tested high quality culture media is now available for purchase from a number of suppliers worldwide, so that media preparation in the laboratory is no longer necessary, and may not be a cost-effective exercise when time and quality control are taken into account.

A list of recommended commercial culture media is supplied at the end of this chapter. There is no scientific evidence that any is superior to another in routine IVF, and choice should depend upon considerations such as quality control and testing procedures applied in its manufacture, cost, and, in particular, guaranteed efficient supply delivery in relation to shelf-life. After delivery, the medium may be aliquoted in suitable smaller volumes, such that one aliquot can be used for a single patient's gamete preparation and culture (including sperm preparation). Media containing HEPES, which maintains a stable pH in the bicarbonate-buffered system, can be used for sperm preparation and oocyte harvesting and washing; however, HEPES is known to alter ion channel activity in the plasma membrane and may well be embryotoxic. The gametes must therefore subsequently be washed in HEPES-free culture medium before insemination and overnight culture. Media specially designated for 'sperm washing' is also commercially available.

Follicular flushing

Ideally, if a patient has responded well to follicular phase stimulation with appropriate monitoring and timing of ovulation induction by human chorionic gonadotrophin (hCG) injection, the oocyte retrieval may proceed smoothly with efficient recovery of oocytes without flushing the follicles. If the number of follicles is low or the procedure is difficult for technical reasons, follicles may be flushed with a physiological solution to assist recovery of all the oocytes present. Balanced salt solutions such as Earle's (EBSS) may be used for follicular flushing, and heparin may be added at a concentration of 2 units/ml. HEPES buffered media can also be used for flushing. Temperature and pH of flushing media must be carefully controlled, and the oocytes recovered from flushing media subsequently washed in culture media before transfer to their final culture droplet or well.

Quality control procedures

The ultimate test of quality control must rest with pregnancy and live birth rates per IVF treatment cycle. An ongoing record of the results of fertilization, cleavage, and embryo development provide the best short-term evidence of good quality control (QC). Daily records in the form of a laboratory log book are essential, summarizing details of patients and outcome of laboratory procedures: age, cause of infertility, stimulation protocol, number of oocytes retrieved, semen analysis, sperm preparation details, insemination time, fertilization, cleavage, embryo transfer, and cryopreservation. It is also essential to record details of media and oil batches for reference, along with the introduction of any new methods or materials used. Although some routine IVF laboratories rely upon a mouse embryo culture system for quality control assurance, the validity of this test has been questioned as a reliable assay for extrapolation to clinical IVF. Any new batches of material or supplies used in the culture system, if not pre-tested, should be tested before use. Suggested QC procedures include the following:

1. Sperm survival test

Select a normal sample of washed prepared spermatozoa and assess for count, motility, and progression. Divide the selected sample into four aliquots: add test material to two aliquots, and equivalent control material (in current use) to 2 aliquots. Incubate one control and one test sample at 37 °C, and one of each at room temperature. Assess each sample for count, motility, and progression after 24 and 48 hours (a computer-aided system can be used if available).

Test and control samples should show equivalent survival. If there is any doubt, repeat the test.

2. Culture of surplus oocytes

Surplus oocytes from patients who have large numbers of oocytes retrieved may be used to test new culture material. Culture at least six oocytes in the control media, and a maximum of four in test media.

3. Multipronucleate embryo culture

Oocytes which show abnormal fertilization on day 1 after insemination can be used for testing new batches of material. Observe, score, and assess each embryo daily until day 6 after insemination.

4. Culture of 'spare' embryos

Surplus embryos after embryo transfer which are not suitable for freezing can also be used for testing new culture material. Observe, score, and assess each embryo daily as above. Embryo development to a normal blastocyst is regarded as evidence of adequate culture conditions, and normal blastocysts may be cryopreserved.

Tissue culture systems

Vessels successfully used for in vitro fertilization include test tubes, four-well culture dishes, organ culture dishes, and petri dishes containing microdroplets of culture medium under a layer of paraffin or mineral oil. Whatever the system employed, it must be capable of rigidly maintaining fixed stable parameters of temperature, pH, and osmolarity. Human oocytes are extremely sensitive to transient cooling in vitro, and modest reductions in temperature can cause irreversible disruption of the meiotic spindle, with possible chromosome dispersal. Analyses of embryos produced by IVF have shown that a high proportion are chromosomally abnormal, and it is possible that temperature-induced chromosome disruption may contribute to the high rates of preclinical and spontaneous abortion that follow IVF and gamete intrafallopian transfer (GIFT). Therefore, it is essential to control temperature fluctuation from the moment of follicle aspiration, and during all oocyte and embryo manipulations, by using heated microscope stages and heating blocks or platforms.

An overlay of equilibrated oil as part of the tissue culture system confers specific advantages:

1. The oil acts as a physical barrier, separating droplets of medium from the atmosphere and air-borne particles or pathogens.
2. Oil prevents evaporation and delays gas diffusion, thereby keeping pH, temperature, and osmolality of the medium stable during gamete manipulations, protecting the embryos from significant fluctuations in their microenvironment.
3. Oil prevents evaporation: humidified and pre-equilibrated oil allows the use of non-humidified incubators, which are easier to clean and maintain.

(It has also been suggested that oil could enhance embryo development by removing lipid-soluble toxins from the medium).

The physical properties of oil result in very slow diffusion of gas through the overlay, so the oil must be prepared and equilibrated in advance. Unequilibrated oil could absorb gas from the media, producing an alkaline pH with adverse effects upon the gametes or embryos.

Oil preparation

Mineral or paraffin oil should be sterile as supplied, and does not require filtration or autoclaving. Equilibrate the oil by adding approximately 100 ml of oil to 20 ml of a balanced salt solution such as Earles (without serum). Bubble 5% CO_2 though the bottle for 5–10 minutes, shake gently, and allow to settle overnight at room temperature before use. This washing procedure removes water-soluble toxins; non-water soluble toxins may also be present which will not be removed by washing, and therefore it is wise to test new batches of oil with, at the very least, sperm survival test as a quality control procedure. Oil overlays should be equilibrated in the CO_2 incubator for several hours before use.

Serum supplements

Commercially prepared media are supplied complete, and do not require the addition of any supplements; most contain a serum substitute such as 'albuminar', human serum albumin. No significant differences have been found in fertilization, cleavage, or pregnancy rates when maternal serum was compared with human serum albumin supplementing culture media; however, development to blastocyst stage may be enhanced when maternal serum is used. If maternal serum is used in the culture system, it must be homologous; pooled or donor sera are not recommended, even after thorough viral screening.

Preparation of maternal serum

Collect 20 ml of the patient's blood by venepuncture, maintain in an ice bucket, and spin immediately, before the sample clots. Remove the supernatant serum, and leave it to clot for approximately 30–60 minutes. Remove the clot by compressing it around a pasteur pipette, and heat inactivate the serum at 56 °C for 45 minutes. Cool, and then filter through two millipore filters of 0.45 µm and 0.22 µm in sequence. Store at 4 °C. Maternal serum must not be used in cases of immunological or idiopathic infertility, or in cases with a previous history of unexplained failed fertilization.

Basic equipment required for the IVF laboratory

Embryology

CO_2 incubator
Dissecting microscope
Inverted microscope
Heated surfaces for microscope and manipulation areas
Heating block for test tubes
Laminar flow cabinet
Oven for heat-sterilizing
Small autoclave
Water bath
Pipette 10–100 µl Eppendorf
Pipette 20–1000 µl Eppendorf
Refrigerator

Supply of 5% CO_2 in air
Wash bottle + Millex filter for gas
Rubber tubing
Pipette canisters
Mineral or paraffin oil
Culture media

Glassware for media preparation
Osmometer (for media preparation)
Weighing balance
Millipore Bell filter unit for filtering media

Tissue culture plastics: (Nunc, Corning, Sterilin)
Flasks for media and oil: 50 ml, 175 ml
Culture dishes: 60, 35 mm
OCR (oocyte retrieval) needles
Test tubes for OCR: 17 ml disposable
Transfer catheters: embryo, GIFT, IUI
Syringes
Needles
Disposable pipettes: 1, 5, 10, 25 ml
'Pipetus' pipetting device
Eppendorf tips, small and large
Millipore filters: 0.22, 0.8 µm
Glass Pasteur pipettes (Volac)
Pipette bulbs
Test tube racks

Spirit burners + methanol or gas Bunsen burner
Rubbish bags
Tissues
Tape for labelling
7X detergent (Flow)
70% ethanol
Sterile gloves

Oil: Boots, Squibb, Sigma, Medicult
Supply of purified water: Milli-Q system or Analar
Glassware for making culture media: beakers, flasks, measuring cylinder

Details of IVF media can be obtained from the following manufacturing companies:

Medicult: Lersø Parkalle 42, Dk-2100 Copenhagen, Denmark
Scandinavian IVF Science AB, Mölndalsvägen 30A, PO Box 14105, Göthenburg, Sweden
Menezo B2: Bio-Merieux, France
Ham's F-10, EBSS: Flow Laboratories, UK
HTF: Irvine Scientific, USA
Bio-Care International, San Diego, CA 92121, USA

Further reading

Almeida, P.A. & Bolton, V.N. (1996) The effect of temperature fluctuations on the cytoskeletal organisation and chromosomal constitution of the human oocyte. *Zygote* **3**: 357–365.

Angell, R.R., Templeton, A.A. & Aitken, R.J. (1986) Chromosome studies in human in vitro fertilisation. *Human Genetics* **72**: 333–339.

Ashwood-Smith, M.J., Hollands, P. & Edwards, R.G., (1989) The use of Albuminar (TM) as a medium supplement in clinical IVF. *Human Reproduction* **4**: 702–705.

Augustus, D. (1996) Cell culture incubators: tips for successful routine maintenance. *Alpha Newsletter* vol.4, April 1996.

Danforth, R.A., Piana, S.D. & Smith, M. (1987) High purity water: an important component for success in in vitro fertilisation. *American Biotechnology Laboratory* **5**: 58–60.

Davidson, A., Vermesh, M., Lobo, R.A. & Paulsen, R.J. (1988) Mouse embryo culture as quality control for human in vitro fertilisation: the one-cell versus two-cell model. *Fertility and Sterility* **49**: 516–521.

Edwards, R.G. & Brody, S.A. (1995) Human fertilization in the laboratory. In: *Principles and Practice of Assisted Human Reproduction*, W.B. Saunders & Co., Philadelphia, Pennsylvania, pp. 351–413.

Fleetham, J. & Mahadevan, M.M. (1988) Purification of water for in vitro fertilization and embryo transfer. *Journal of In Vitro Fertilization and Embryo Transfer* **5**: 171–147.

Fleming, T.P., Pratt, H.P.M. & Braude, P.R. (1987) The use of mouse preimplantation embryos for quality control of culture reagents in human in vitro fertilization programs: a cautionary note. *Fertility and Sterility* **47**: 858–860.

George, M.A., Braude, P.R. & Johnson, M.H., Sweetnam, D.G. (1989) Quality control in the IVF laboratory: in vitro and in vivo development of mouse embryos is unaffected by the quality of water used in culture media. *Human Reproduction* **4**: 826–831.

Johnson, C., Hofmann, G. & Scott, R. (1994) The use of oil overlay for in vitro fertilization and culture. *Assisted Reproduction Review* **4**: 198–201.

Ma, S., Kalousek, D.K., Zouves, C., Yuen, B.H., Gomel, V. & Moon, Y.S. (1990) The chromosomal complements of cleaved human embryos resulting from in vitro fertilization. *Journal of In Vitro Fertilization and Embryo Transfer* **7**: 16–21.

Marrs, R.P., Saito, H., Yee, B., Sato, F. & Brown, J. (1984) Effect of variation of in vitro culture techniques upon oocyte fertilization and embryo development in human in vitro fertilization procedures. *Fertility and Sterility* **41**: 519–523.

Mortimer, D. & Quinn, P. (1996) Bicarbonate-buffered media and CO_2. *Alpha Newsletter* vol. 4, April 1996.

Naaktgeboren, N. (1987) Quality control of culture media for in vitro fertilization. *In Vitro fertilization program*, Academic Hospital, Vrije Universiteit, Brussels, Belgium. *Annal Biologie Clinique (Paris)* **45**: 368–372.

Pellestor, F., Girardet, A., Andreo, B., Arnal, F. & Humeau, C. (1994) Relationship between morphology and chromosomal constitution in human preimplantation embryos. *Molecular and Reproductive Development* **39**: 141–146.

Pickering, S.J., Braude, P.R., Johnson, M.H., Cant, A. & Currie, J. (1990) Transient cooling to room temperature can cause irreversible disruption of the meiotic spindle in the human oocyte. *Fertility and Sterility* **54**: 102–108.

Plachot, M., de Grouchy, J., Montagut, J., Lepetre, S., Carle, E., Veiga, A., Calderon, G. & Santalo, J. (1987) Multicentric study of chromosome analysis in human oocytes and embryos in an IVF programme *Human Reproduction* **2**: 29.

Purdy, J. (1982) Methods for fertilization and embryo culture in vitro. In: *Human Conception In Vitro*, Edwards, R.G. & Purdy, J.M. eds. Academic Press, London, p. 135.

Quinn, P., Warner, G.M., Klein, J.F. & Kirby, C. (1985) Culture factors affecting the success rate of in vitro fertilization and embryo transfer. *Annals of the New York Academy of Sciences* **412**: 195.

Rinehart, J.S., Bavister, B.D. & Gerrity, M. (1988). Quality control in the in vitro fertilization laboratory: comparison of bioassay systems for water quality *Journal of In Vitro Fertilization and Embryo Transfer* **5**: 335–342.

Staessen, C., Van den Abbeel, E., Carle, M., Khan, I., Devroey, P. & Van Steirteghen, A.C. (1990) Comparison between human serum and Albuminar-20(TM) supplement for in vitro fertilization. *Human Reproduction* **5**: 336–341.

Wales, R.G. (1970) Effect of ions on the development of preimplantation mouse embryos in vitro. *Australian Journal of Biological Sciences* **23**: 421–429.

Yovich, J.L., Edirisinghe, W., Yovich, J.M., Stanger, J. & Matson, P. (1988) Methods of water purification for the preparation of culture media in an IVF-ET programme *Human Reproduction* **3**: 245–248.

9
Semen analysis and preparation for assisted reproductive techniques

At least 50% of couples referred for infertility investigation and treatment are found to have a contributing male factor. Male factor infertility can represent a variety of defects, which result in abnormal sperm number, morphology, or function. Detailed analysis of sperm assessment and function are important for accurate diagnosis, and are described in detail in numerous textbooks of practical andrology and semen analysis. A comprehensive review of semen analysis is beyond the scope of this book, and only details relevant to assisted conception treatment will be described here.

The World Health Organization (WHO) laboratory manual describes standard conditions for the collection of semen samples, their delivery, and the standardization of laboratory assessment procedures. The WHO standards indicate that a 'normal' semen sample contains at least 20×10^6 spermatozoa/ml, with at least 50% exhibiting good to excellent forward progressive movement within 60 minutes after ejaculation. The recent introduction of intracytoplasmic sperm injection (ICSI) now provides effective in vitro fertilization (IVF) treatment for even the most severe cases of male infertility which were previously felt to be beyond hope, and the fact that fertilization can be achieved from semen with 'hopeless' sperm parameters has forced a review of standard semen analysis and sperm function testing. This chapter will address only the basic principles required in the practical features of sperm preparation procedures for assisted conception techniques.

Semen assessment

Collection of semen samples

The male partner must be provided with a clearly labelled standard sterile disposable plastic pot. Re-usable glass containers must NOT be used (certain types of glass are toxic, and residues of detergent used for washing are also toxic). The time of sample collection should be clearly recorded on the label. An accompanying form may be completed, describing details of length of abstinence, recent illness, medication taken, smoking, and alcohol consumption.

Samples previously assessed as having high viscosity benefit from collection into pots containing 1 ml of medium. In cases of immunological infertility, when the mixed antiglobulin reaction (MAR), immunobead, or tray agglutination test (TAT) tests indicate the presence of antisperm antibodies in the semen, the sample should be collected into medium containing 50% serum albumin. Immediate processing of these samples on a buoyant density gradient helps to minimize antibody binding to sperm.

Liquefaction

Allow the specimen to liquefy naturally on the bench; liquefaction should be complete within 30 minutes. Before proceeding with the analysis, mix the specimen thoroughly; note and record the colour, and whether the sample runs freely on pipetting. Viscous samples are difficult to pipette, leaving sticky strands. High viscosity will interfere with accurate assessment of motility and density, and repeated aspiration through a pipette or needle can help to break down the viscosity.

Measure the volume using a graduated pipette or syringe

Assessment of density and motility

Accurate asessments of sperm density can be calculated using a haemocytometer to count a sample of immobilized sperm; however, when the purpose of assessment is the selection of an appropriate method of preparing the sample for assisted conception procedures, it may be practical to use a method which allows simultaneous judgment of motile and immotile concentrations, as well as type of sperm motility. Fixed-depth counting chambers (Makler, Horwell, or disposable chambers) allow simultaneous assessment of density and motility in order to choose the most appropriate method of sperm preparation. Place the required sample volume on the chamber, according to the manufacturer's instructions, and examine microscopically using a x 20 objective. Before performing the count, note the following features of the specimen:

    a) The presence of debris and cells other than spermatozoa, such as red or white blood cells

    b) agglutination of spermatoza and type if present (H-H, T-T, H-T)

Examine the counting grid and count the number of *motile* sperm in 20 squares. If the count appears on initial observation to be less than 10 million/ml, all 100 squares should be counted. Count the *total* number of sperm in the same group of squares, and calculate motility :

Sperm density in millions/ml = the number of sperm in 10 squares of the grid.
Motility = No. of motile sperm in $\underline{n}$ number of squares $\times$ 100 divided by total number of sperm in $\underline{n}$ squares

Progression

Progression is assessed on a scale of 0–4 (The Macleod Scale)

- 0 immotile sperm
- 1 motile sperm with no progressive forward movement
- 2 slow forward progressive movement
- 3 moderate forward progressive movement
- 4 rapid, regular forward progression

Morphology

A normal, fertile semen sample contains a very high proportion of morphologically abnormal forms, and the significance of abnormal sperm morphology is not entirely understood. Detailed morphology assessment is carried out by counting a stained slide preparation using bright-field optics at 1000 magnification as described in the WHO manual. Figure 9.1 shows examples of sperm morphology, with measurements of the various components of a normal sperm cell. The normal head has an oval shape with a length:width ratio of 1.50:1.75. A well defined acrosomal region should cover 40–70% of the head area. No neck, midpiece, or tail defects should be evident, and cytoplasmic droplets should constitute no more than one-third the size of a normal sperm head. All borderline forms are classified as abnormal.

Mix a drop of semen on a slide with a drop of 1% formaldehyde in 0.01 mol/L phosphate buffer, and stain with 1% eosin in distilled water followed by 10% nigrosin in distilled water. Cover with a cover slip, and count 200 sperm with a scoring system according to strict Kruger criteria:
(Pre-stained slides are also available: Blustain, Irvine Scientific)

1) Abnormal heads
2) Tail abnormality
3) Midpiece abnormalities
4) Immature forms.

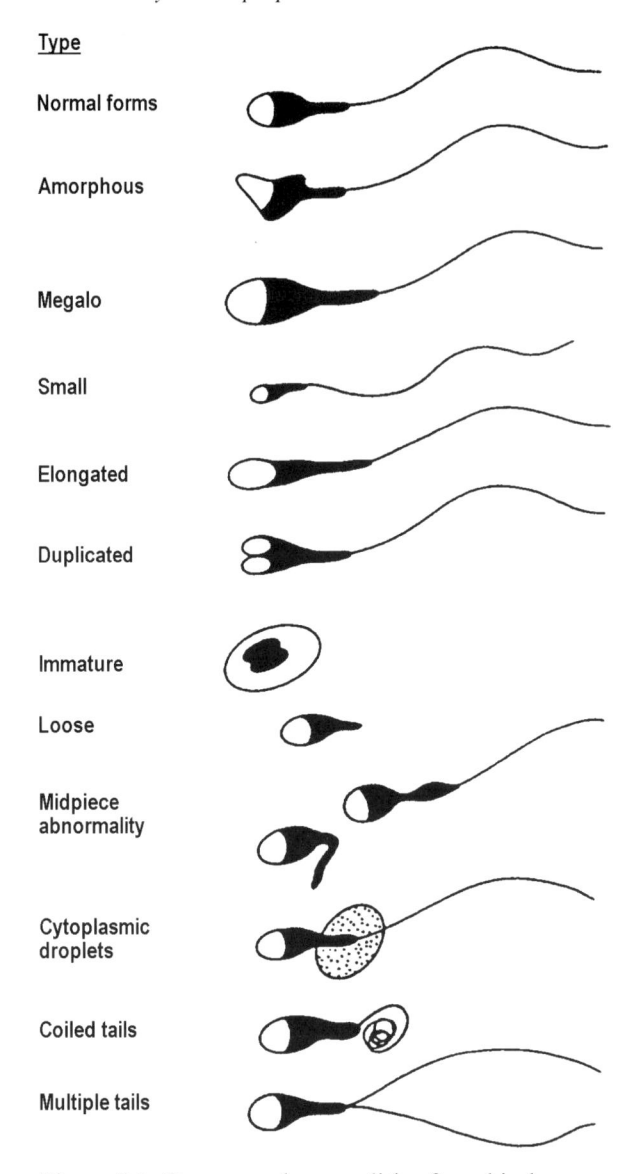

Figure 9.1 Common abnormalities found in human sperm morphology.

Calculate the percentage of each abnormal form, and add together the percentages to yield the total percentage of abnormal forms in the sample.

Mixed antiglobulin reaction (The MAR test)

The MAR test offers a rapid and simple screening test for antisperm antibodies, which can be performed as part of the routine semen analysis. Advance knowledge of the presence of antisperm antibodies can significantly improve

Preparation of sperm for IVF, GIFT and intrauterine insemination 89

the outcome of fertilization by allowing appropriate steps to be taken in sample collection and preparation which will decrease the binding of antibodies to the sperm and thus facilitate fertilization.

Preparation of red blood cells (RBCs)

1. Collect 2 ml of O-positive venous blood by venepuncture and centrifuge at high speed for 15 minutes.
2. Aspirate the serum from the separated RBCs.
3. Add an equivalent amount of Alsevers solution (Gibco, cat. no. 04305190M) to the RBCs, mix and centrifuge again for 15 minutes.
4. Aspirate the clear solution, and add the same volume of Alsevers solution. Centrifuge, and repeat the washing procedure twice.
5. Remove the clear solution, add 1/5 volume of anti-D to RBCs (approx volume of anti-D=1/5 volume of RBCs). Mix and incubate at 37 °C for 30 minutes.
6. Add an equivalent volume of Alsevers solution to RBCs, centrifuge again for 15 minutes and repeat again twice, aspirating clear solution after each centrifugation.
7. Add enough Alsevers solution to washed RBCs to give a final haematocrit of 5–10% (i.e. to 1 ml of RBCs add 10 ml Alsevers solution).

MAR Test

The semen sample to be tested must have a count $>5\times 10^6$/ml, and motility $>10\%$

1. Add one drop of O-positive sensitized blood to one drop semen and mix thoroughly.
2. Add one drop anti-IgG solution. Mix.
3. Place a coverslip over the mixture, leave for 3 minutes, and then assess.
4. Shaking movements of RBCs indicate a positive reaction, i.e. antisperm antibodies are present. The reaction will show variable positive reactions.
5. The RBCs will clump normally. Only clumps whose shaking is due to bound motile spermatozoa indicate a positive reaction

    += <50% of sperms bound
   ++= 50% of sperms bound
 +++= virtually all sperms bound

Preparation of sperm for in vitro fertilization/GIFT/intrauterine insemination

At the time of oocyte retrieval or intrauterine insemination (IUI), the laboratory should already be familiar with the male partner's semen profile, and can refer to features which might influence the choice of sperm preparation method used. The choice of sperm preparation method or combination of methods depends upon the assessment of:

- the motile count
- ratio between motile: immotile count
- volume
- presence of antibodies, agglutination, pus cells or debris

Sterile technique must be used throughout

Ejaculated semen is a viscous liquid composed of a mixture of testicular and epididymal secretions containing spermatozoa, mixed with prostatic secretions produced at the time of ejaculation. This seminal plasma contains substances which inhibit capacitation and prevent fertilization. The purpose of sperm preparation is to concentrate the motile spermatozoa in a fraction which is free of seminal plasma and its debris. Although sperm can be prepared by simple washing and centrifugation, the method applied to early IVF practice, this method also concentrates cells, debris, and immotile sperm, the presence of which jeopardizes fertilization. Aitken *et al.* (1987) have demonstrated that white cells and dead sperm in semen are a source of reactive oxygen species which can initiate lipid peroxidation in human sperm membranes. Peroxidation of sperm membrane unsaturated fatty acids leads to a loss of membrane fluidity, which inhibits sperm fusion events during the process of fertilization. When preparing sperm for asssisted conception it is advantageous to separate motile sperm from leucocytes and dead sperm as effectively and efficiently as possible.

Sperm samples which show moderate to high counts ($>35\times10^6$ motile sperm/ml) with good forward progression and motility can be prepared using a basic overlay and swim-up technique. Discontinuous buoyant density gradient centrifugation is the method of choice for samples which show:

1. Low motility
2. Poor forward progression
3. Large amounts of debris and/or high numbers of cells
4. Antisperm antibodies

At the end of each preparation procedure, the pH of the resulting samples is adjusted by gassing gently with 5% CO_2, and samples are stored at room temperature until final preparation for insemination.

Standard swim-up or layering

Pipette 2 ml of culture medium into a 10 ml round-bottomed disposable test tube. Gently pipette approximately 1.5 ml neat semen underneath the medium (being very careful not to disturb the interface formed between the semen and the medium). Tightly cap the tube and allow it to stand at room temperature for up to 2 hours. The ejaculate can also be divided into several tubes for layering if necessary. Harvest the resulting top and middle clouded layers into a conical test tube and spin at 200 g for 5 minutes. Remove the supernatant and resuspend the pellet in 2 ml medium. Centrifuge again, discard the supernatant, and resuspend the pellet in 1 ml medium. Assess this sample for count and motility, gas the surface gently with 5% CO_2 in air, and store at room temperature prior to dilution for the insemination procedure.

Alternatively, 2 ml of medium can be gently layered over the semen sample in its pot, which provides a larger interface surface area. After 10–45 minutes, suspend an aliquot of this layer in 1 ml of medium, and process as above.

The time allowed for swim-up should be adjusted according to the quality of the initial sample: the percentage of abnormal sperm which will appear in the medium increases with time, and continues to do so after normal motile density has reached its optimum level.

Pellet and swim-up

This method is used when the semen has been collected into medium or medium + serum. It is also useful for viscous samples (once the viscosity has been decreased, by vigorous pipetting or syringing) and when the total volume of semen is very low. This method is not recommended when motility is very poor or when there is a large degree of cellular contamination and debris (the sperm will be concentrated with this prior to the swim-up).

1. Mix semen and medium and centrifuge once.
   N.B. In some cases (i.e. oligo/asthenospermia) much more semen will need to be prepared, and the volume of medium used should be increased accordingly. As a general rule be careful not to take far more of the semen than is required.
2. Carefully remove all the supernatant and then very gently pipette about 0.75 ml of medium over the pellet, taking care not to disturb it.
3. Allow the sperm to swim-up into the medium. If the sample has poor motility it sometimes helps to lay the centrifuge tube on its side.
   – 10 minutes is sufficient for very motile sperm (activity 3–4)
   – 1 hour plus may be required for poorly motile sperm.
   In general do not leave for too long, as some cells and debris will become resuspended.
4. Carefully remove supernatant from pellet and place in a clean centrifuge tube.
5. Centrifuge again, resuspend in medium, assess count and motility, and gas with CO_2 before storing at room temperature.

This method has the disadvantage of exposing motile sperm to peroxidative damage during centrifugation with defective sperm and white cells. Aitken (1990) has shown that unselected sperm exhibit higher levels of reactive oxygen species production in response to centrifugation than the functionally competent sperm selected prior to centrifugation by the layering method. Sperm that are selected prior to centrifugation produce much lower levels of reactive oxygen species, and their functional capacity is not impaired.

Discontinuous bouyant density gradient centrifugation

A suspension of silica particles coated with polyvinylpyrrolidone, can be used to create buoyant density gradients for sperm preparation. Buoyant density apparently protects the sperm from the trauma of centrifugation, and a high proportion of functional sperm can be recovered from the gradients. Discontinuous two- or three-step gradients are simple to prepare and highly effective in preparing motile sperm fractions from suboptimal semen samples.

Methods

The following 'recipes' should be adapted according to each individual semen sample, in particular with respect to volumes, speed of centrifugation, and length of centrifugation. In general, a longer centrifugation *time* increases the recovery of both motile and immotile sperm; normal immotile sperm are only decelerated by the particles, and after long spinning they will reach the bottom of the gradient. Higher centrifugation *speeds* increase the recovery of motile sperm, and also of lower density particles; therefore, if the gradients are spun at a higher speed, a shorter time should be used. Debris, round cells, and abnormal forms with amorphous heads and cytoplasmic droplets never reach the bottom of the tube because of their low density. Gradients with larger volumes result in improved filtration, but decreased yield. The three layers of a mini-gradient improve filtration, and the smaller volumes improve recovery of sperm from severely oligospermic samples. Large amounts of debris can disrupt gradients and prevent adequate filtration. Samples with a large amount of debris should be distributed in smaller volumes over several gradients. Severely asthenozoospermic samples, with a normal sperm density but poor motility can also be distributed over a series of mini-gradients.

Isotonic gradient solution

10 × concentrated EBS (or other media concentrate)	10 ml
5% human serum albumin	9 ml
Sodium pyruvate	3 mg
Sodium lactate @ 60%	0.37 ml
1 M HEPES	2 ml
Gentamicin sulphate, 5 mg/ml	2 ml

Mix, and filter this solution through a 0.22 μm Millipore filter,

> Add 90 ml density gradient preparation
> Store at +4 °C for up to 1 week

Two-step gradient, 80/40

Can be used for all samples which contain more than four million motile sperm/ml. Should be used for all specimens with known or suspected antisperm antibodies

> 80%: 8 ml isotonic + 2 ml culture medium
> 40%: 4 ml isotonic + 6 ml culture medium

1. Gradients: pipette 2.0–2.5 ml of 80% into the bottom of a conical centrifuge tube.
   Gently overlay with an equal volume of 40%.
   Layer up to 2 ml of sample on top of the 40% layer.
2. Centrifuge at 600 g for 20 minutes.
   Cells, debris, and immotile/abnormal sperm accumulate at the interfaces, and the pellet should contain functionally normal sperm. Recovery of a good pellet is influenced by the amount of debris and immotile sperm which impede the travel of the good sperm.
3. Carefully recover the pellet at the bottom of the 80% layer, resuspend in 1 ml of medium, and assess (even if there is no visible pellet, a sufficient number of sperm can usually be recovered by aspirating the bottom 20–50 μl of the 80% layer).
4. If the sample looks sufficiently clean, centrifuge for 5 minutes at 200 g, resuspend the pellet in fresh medium, and assess the final preparation.
5. If there is a high percentage of immotile sperm, centrifuge at 200 g for 5 minutes, remove the supernatant, carefully layer 1 ml fresh medium over the pellet, and allow the motile sperm to swim up for 15–30 minutes.
   Collect the supernatant and assess the final preparation.

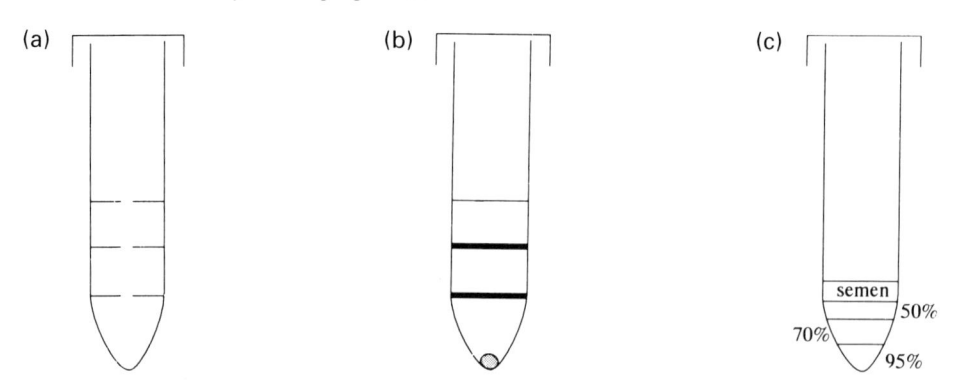

Figure 9.2 Buoyant density gradients. (a, b) Two-step gradients before and after centrifugation; (c) Mini-gradient.

If at least 10^6 motile sperm/ml have been recovered, spin at 200 g for 5 minutes and resuspend in fresh medium. This will be the final preparation to be diluted before insemination, therefore the volume of medium added will depend upon the calculated assessment.

Mini-gradient (95/70/50)

95%	9.5 ml Percoll	+ 0.5 ml culture medium
70%	7.0 ml	3.0 ml
50%	5.0 ml	5.0 ml

1. Gradients: make layers with 0.3 ml of each solution: 95, then 70, then 50.
2. Dilute the semen 1:1 with culture medium, and centrifuge at 200 g for 10 minutes.
3. Resuspend the pellet in 0.3 ml culture medium, and layer over mini-gradient (resuspend in a larger volume if it is to be distributed over several gradients)
4. Centrifuge at 600 g, 20–30 minutes.
5. Recover the pellet(s), resuspend in 0.5 ml culture medium, and assess count and motility. Proceed exactly as for two-step gradient preparation: either centrifuge at 200 g for 5 minutes and resuspend the pellet, or layer over the pellet for a further preparation by swim up. The concentration of the final preparation should be adjusted to a sperm density of approximately one million motile sperm per ml if possible (Figure 9.2).

NB: if a sample is being prepared for ICSI, note that residual PVP-coated particles in the preparation will interact with polyvinylpyrrolidone (PVP), resulting in a gelatinous mass from which the sperm cannot be aspirated!! *Careful washing of the preparation to remove all traces of gradient preparation is essential when handling samples for ICSI.*

Sedimentation method or layering under paraffin oil

This method is useful for samples with very low counts and poor motility. It is very effective in removing debris, but requires several hours of preparation time.

1. Mix the semen with a large volume of medium, pipetting thoroughly to break down viscosity etc. and wash the sample by dilution and centrifugation twice.
2. Alternatively: process the entire sample (undiluted) on an appropriate discontinuous buoyant density gradient.
3. Resuspend the pellet in a reduced volume of medium so that the final motile sperm concentration is not too dilute.
4. Layer this final suspension under paraffin oil (making one large droplet) in a small petri dish. Place in a desiccator and gas with 5% CO_2.
5. Leave at room temperature for 3–24 hours. The duration of sedimentation depends upon the amount of cells, debris and motile spermatozoa; a longer period is usually more effective in reducing cells and debris, but may also reduce the number of freely motile sperm in the upper part of the droplet.
6. Carefully aspirate motile sperm by pipetting the upper part of the droplet. Aspiration can be made more efficient by using a fine drawn pipette and also by positioning the droplet under the stereomicroscope, to ensure that as little debris as possible is collected.

High-speed centrifugation and washing

Cryptozoospermic (or nearly cryptozoospermic) samples which must be prepared for ICSI can be either centrifuged directly (without dilution) at 1800 g for 5 minutes, or diluted with medium and then centrifuged at 1800 g for 5 minutes.

Wash the pellet with a small volume of medium (0.5 ml approximately) and centrifuge at 200 g for 5 minutes. Recover this pellet in a minimal volume of medium (20–50 µl), and overlay with mineral oil. Single sperm for microinjection can then be retrieved from this droplet using the micromanipulator.

It is important to bear in mind that every semen specimen has different characteristics and parameters, and it is illogical to treat each specimen identically. All preparation methods are adaptable in some way: layering can be carried out in test tubes, but a wider vessel increases the area exposed to culture medium and decreases the depth of the specimen, increasing the potential return of motile sperm from oligoasthenospermic samples. Centrifugation times for buoyant density gradients may be adjusted according to the quality of the specimen to give optimum results. It is important to tailor preparation techniques to fit the parameters of the semen specimen, rather than to have fixed recipes. A trial preparation prior to oocyte retrieval may be advisable in choosing the suitable technique for particular patients.

Methods of sperm preparation

- Overlay and swim-up, multiple overlay
- Discontinuous buoyant density gradients
    - mini: 95/70/50%
    - two-step: 40/80, 45/90, 47.5/95%
    - one-step: 95%
- High-speed centrifugation and washing
    - sedimentation under oil
    - 'fishing' with micromanipulator
    - swim-out under oil

Be flexible: use and adapt a combination of methods

Chemical enhancement of sperm motility prior to insemination

Pentoxifylline is a methyl-xanthine derived phosphodiesterase inhibitor which is known to elevate spermatozoal intracellular levels of cyclic adenosine 3´5´ monophosphate in vitro. It has been postulated that the resulting increase in intracellular adenosine triphosphate (ATP) enhances sperm motility in samples which on assessment show poor progressive motility, with an increase in fertilization and pregnancy rates for suboptimal semen samples. 2–Deoxyadenosine has also been used to achieve a similar effect.

The protocol involves a 30 minute preincubation of prepared sperm with the stimulant; the resulting sperm suspension is then washed to remove the stimulant, and the preparation is used immediately for insemination.

Stock solutions:

1 mM PF: dissolve 22 mg Pentoxifylline (Hoechst) in 10 ml medium
3 mM 2-DA: dissolve 8 mg 2–deoxyadenosine in 10 ml medium
Gas with 5% CO_2 to adjust pH
Store at 4 °C for a maximum period of one month

Procedure:

1. Gas and warm PF or 2-DA solutions, and also an additional 10 ml medium
2. 35–40 minutes prior to insemination time, add an equal volume of PF or 2-DA solutions to the sperm preparation suspension

3. Incubate at 37 °C for 30 minutes.
4. Centrifuge, 5 minutes, 200 g, and resuspend pellet in warm medium.
5. Analyse the sperm suspension for count and motility, dilute to appropriate concentration for insemination, and inseminate oocytes immediately.

Sperm preparation for ICSI

A combination of sperm preparation methods can be used:

Extremely oligospermic/asthenozoospermic samples cannot be prepared by buoyant density centrifugation or swim-up techniques.

1. Centrifuge the whole sample, 1800 g, 5 minutes, wash with medium, and resuspend the pellet in a small volume of medium.
2. Apply this sample directly to the injection dish, without PVP, or add an aliquot of the suspension to a drop of HEPES buffered medium without PVP.
3. If possible, use the injection pipette to select a moving sperm with apparently normal morphology from this drop, and transfer it into the PVP drop.
4. If there is debris attached to the sperm, clean it by pipetting the sperm back and forth with the injection pipette.
5. If the sperm still has some movement in the PVP drop, immobilize it and proceed with the injection as previously described.
6. It may sometimes be helpful to connect the sperm droplet to another small medium droplet by means of a bridge of medium, and allow motile sperm to swim out into the clean droplet.

Obstructive azoospermia: epididymal and testicular sperm

1. Epididymal sperm can be obtained by open microscopic surgery or by percutaneous puncture, using a 21 g "butterfly" or equivalent needle to aspirate fluid.
   If large numbers of sperm are found, they can be processed by buoyant density gradient centrifugation or even by swim-up techniques. If only a few sperm are found, the sample may be put into drops under oil, and washed in medium drops using the micromanipulator.
2. Testicular sperm can also be obtained by open biopsy or by percutaneous needle biopsy. The specimen obtained is crushed gently between two microscope slides, and the sample then layered on an appropriate buoyant density gradient as per the routine protocol. If there are very few sperm cells after crushing the specimen, single cells may be selected from the specimen using the micromanipulator.

Epididymal and testicular sperm may often be sticky. They have approximately equal fertilizing capacity, which seems to be slightly lower than that of ejaculated sperm. If an adequate number of sperm is recovered during any of the operative procedures, cryopreservation is strongly recommended. Fertilization can be achieved with ICSI using frozen-thawed epididymal and testicular sperm.

No motile sperm

Even if the results of semen analysis have shown no motile sperm to be present, it may be possible to see occasional slight tail movement in a medium drop without PVP. If absolutely no motile sperm are found, immotile sperm may be used. The fertilization rate with immotile sperm is generally lower than that with motile sperm, and oocytes with a single pronucleus are seen more often in these cases. Previous assessment with a vital stain may be helpful before deciding upon ICSI treatment.

100% abnormal heads

If the semen analysis shows 100% head anomalies, it may still be possible to find the occasional normal form in the sample. In cases where no normal forms are found, the fertilization and implantation rates may be lower; however, debate continues about this subject, and individual judgment should be applied to each case, with careful assessment of several different semen samples.

Fertilization and pregnancy have now been demonstrated using samples from men with globozoospermia, a 100% head anomaly where all sperm lack an acrosomal cap; however, recent evidence suggests that such defects which are genetically determined have a high probability of being transmitted to the offspring, and debate continues as to whether it is ethically advisable to offer treatment to these men.

Sticky Sperm

Sperm which have a tendency to stick to the injection pipette make the injection procedure more difficult. If the sperm is caught in the pipette, try to release it by repeatedly aspirating and blowing with the injection system.

Excessive amounts of debris

Large amounts of debris in the sperm preparation may block the injection pipette, or become attached to the outside of the pipette. A blocked pipette may be cleared by blowing a small amount of the air already in the pipette through it (or by using 'Sonic Sword' from Research Instruments). Debris attached to the outside of the injection pipette can be cleaned by rubbing the pipette against the holding pipette, against the oocyte, or against the oil at the edge of the medium drop. It may be necessary (and preferable) to change the pipette if it cannot be quickly cleared.

Retrograde ejaculation and electroejaculation: sperm preparation

When treating patients with ejaculatory dysfunction, with or without the aid of electroejaculation, both antegrade and retrograde ejaculation (into the bladder) are commonly found. When retrograde ejaculation is anticipated, the bladder should first be emptied via a catheter, and approximately 20 ml of culture medium then instilled. After ejaculation, the bladder is again emptied, and the entire sample centrifuged. The resulting pellet(s) can then be resuspended in medium and processed on appropriate density gradients. As with all abnormal semen samples, a flexible approach is required in order to obtain a suitable sample for insemination.

Sperm preparation: equipment and materials

Semen sterile collection pot 60 ml
Microscope (phase is useful)
Counting chamber (Makler, Sefi Medical Instruments, POB 7295, Haifa 31070 Israel, or Horwell Haemocytometer)
Centrifuge with swing-out rotor (Mistral 1000, MSE)
Centrifuge tubes (15 ml, Corning)
Microscope slides
Coverslips
Disposable test tubes: 4ml, 10 ml
Culture media
Buoyant Density Media:
    Pure Sperm (Scandinavian IVF AB)
    MediCult Percoll Medium
    Sil-Select (MICROM)
    Isolate (Irvine Scientific)
Glass Pasteur pipettes
Disposable pipettes: 1, 5, 10 ml
Spirit burner + methanol or gas Bunsen burner
Plastic ampoules or straws for sperm freezing
Sperm cryopreservation media (Chapter 11)
Supply of liquid nitrogen and storage Dewars

Further reading

Aitken, R.J. (1988) Assessment of sperm funtion for IVF. *Human Reproduction* **3**: 89–95.

Aitken, R.J. (1989) The role of free oxygen radicals and sperm function. *International Journal of Andrology* **12**: 95–97

Aitken, R.J. & Clarkson, J.S. (1987) Cellular basis of defective sperm function and its association with the genesis of reactive oxygen species by human spermatozoa. *Journal of Reproductive Fertility* **81**: 459–469.

Aitken, R.J., Comhaire, F.H., Eliasson, R., Jager, S., Kremer, J., Jones W.R., de Kretscr, D.M., Nieschlag, G., Paulse, C.A., Wang, C. & Waites, G.M.H. *WHO Manual for the Examination of Human Semen and Semen:Cervical Mucus Interaction*, second edition, Cambridge University Press, Cambridge, England, 1987.

Aitken, R.J. (1990) Evaluation of human sperm function. *British Medical Bulletin* **46**: 654–764.

Avery, S.M. & Elder, K.T. (1992) Semen assessment and preparation. In: *In Vitro Fertilization and Assisted Reproduction*, (Brinsden, P.R., Rainsbury, P.A. eds), The Parthenon Publishing Group, UK, pp.171–185.

Avery, S.M., Marriott, V., Mason, B., Riddle, A. & Sharma, V. (1987) An assessment of the efficiency of various sperm preparation techniques. Presented at Vth World Congress on IVF and ET, *Programme Supplement* **85**: p. 58.

Braude, P.R. & Bolton, V.N. (1984) The preparation of spermatozoa for in vitro fertilization by buoyant density centrifugation. In: *Recent Progress in Human In Vitro Fertilization* (Feichtinger, W., Kemeter, P. eds), Cofese, Palermo, pp. 125–134.

Cohen, J., Edwards, R.G., Fehilly, C., Fishel, S., Hewitt, J., Purdy, J., Rowland, G., Steptoe, P.C. & Webster, J. (1985) In vitro fertilization: a treatment for male infertility. *Fertility and Sterility* **43**: 422–432.

Comhaire, F., Depoorter, B,. Vermeulen, L. & Schoonjans, F. (1995) Assessment of sperm concentration. In: *Fertility & Sterility: A Current Overview (IFFS-95)* (Hedon, P. Binger, P. Mares, eds), The Parthenon Publishing Group, New York, London, pp. 297–302.

Dravland, J.E. & Mortimer, D. (1985) A simple discontinuous Percoll gradient for washing human spermatozoa. *IRCS Medical Science* **13**: 16–18.

Elder, K.T., Wick, K.L. & Edwards, R.G. (1990) Seminal plasma anti-sperm antibodies and IVF: the effect of semen sample collection into 50% serum. *Human Reproduction* **5**: 179–184.

Edwards, R.G., Fishel, S.G., Cohen, J., Fehilly, C.B., Purdy, J.M., Steptoe, P.C. & Webster, J.M. (1984) Factors influencing the success of in vitro fertilization for alleviating human infertility. *Journal of In Vitro Fertilization and Embryo Transfer* **1**: 3–23.

Glover, T.D., Barratt, C.L.R., Tyler, J.P.A. & Hennessey, J.F. (1990) *Human male fertility and semen analysis.* Academic Press, London.

Hall, J., Fishel, S., Green, S., Fleming, S., Hunter, A., Stoddart, N., Dowell, K. & Thornton, S. (1995) Intracytoplasmic sperm injection versus high insemination concentration in-vitro fertilization in cases of very severe teratozoospermia. *Human Reproduction* **10**: 493–496.

Jager, S., Kremer, J. & Van-Schlochteren-Draaisma, T. (1978) A simple method of screening for antisperm antibodies in the human male: detection of spermatozoa surface IgG with the direct mixed antiglobulin reaction carried out on untreated fresh human semen. *International Journal of Fertility* **23**: 12–21.

Makler, A. (1978) A new chamber for rapid sperm count and motility evaluation. *Fertility and Sterility* **30:** 313–318.

Menkveld, R., Oettler, E.E., Kruger, T.F., Swanson, R.J., Acosta, A.A. & Oehninger, S. (1991) *Atlas of Human Sperm Morphology*. Williams & Wilkins, Baltimore, MD.

Mortimer, D. (1991) Sperm preparation techniques and iatrogenic failures of in-vitro fertilization. *Human Reproduction* **6:** 173–176.

Mortimer, D. (1994) *Practical Laboratory Andrology*. Oxford University Press, New York.

Rainsbury, P.A. (1992) The treatment of male factor infertility due to sexual dysfunction. In: *In Vitro Fertilization and Assisted Reproduction* (P.R. Brinsden, P.A. Rainsbury, eds), The Parthenon Publishing Group, UK.

Van der Ven, H., Bhattacharya, A.K. Binor, Z., Leto, S. & Zaneveld, L.J.D. (1982) Inhibition of human sperm capacitation by a high molecular weight factor from human seminal plasma. *Fertility and Sterility* **38:** 753–755.

World Health Organization (1992) *WHO Laboratory manual for the examination of human semen and semen-cervical mucus interaction*. Cambridge University Press, Cambridge.

Yovich, J.L. (1992) Assisted reproduction for male factor infertility. In: *In Vitro Fertilization and Assisted Reproduction* (P.R. Brinsden, P.A. Rainsbury, eds), The Parthenon Publishing Group, UK.

Yovich, J.M., Edirisinghe, W.R., Cummins, J.M. & Yovich, J.L. (1990) Influence of pentoxifylline in severe male factor infertility. *Fertility and Sterility* **53:** 715–722.

10
Oocyte retrieval and embryo culture

Programmed superovulation protocols

Programmed superovulation protocols now provide a convenient and effective means of scheduling and organising a clinical IVF programme, allowing oocyte retrievals to be done on specific days of the week, or in 'batches'. The standard protocol used at Bourn Hall to maximize the number of oocytes recovered uses downregulation with gonadotrophin releasing hormone (GnRH) agonist, commencing in the luteal phase of the previous cycle, and ovarian stimulation with purified follicular stimulating hormone (FSH) (Metrodin HP or Gonal F, Serono Laboratorie, UK) by subcutaneous injection.

Protocol

1. Commence downregulation on day 19–21 of the cycle, depending upon menstrual history and cycle length. Rx: nafarelin (Synarel, Searle) two sniffs (400 mg twice daily), or buserelin (Suprefact, Hoechst) 500 mg subcutaneously daily.
2. Programmed cycles allow for 6–12 days of stimulation, varied according to the individual patient's age, cause of infertility, and previous history.
3. Before starting follicular stimulation: confirm downregulation with baseline assessments
    - ultrasound pelvic scan
    - plasma assays for oestrogen, luteinizing hormone (LH), and progesterone.

    If any of the endocrine parameters are elevated (oestradiol (E2) >50 ng/ml, LH >5.0 IU/ml, P4 >2.0 ng/ml), stimulation is postponed and the assays repeated after 2–4 further days of downregulation.
4. Standard starting dose of gonadotropin for stimulation = two or three ampoules daily, varied according to age of patient and previous history, etc. Polycystic ovary (PCO) patients start with one ampoule, and are carefully monitored.
5. Ovulation is induced by subcutaneous administration of human chorionic

Drug treatment for scheduled cycles

- Pituitary downregulation with GnRH agonist: Synarel(Syntex) by intranasal administration, twice daily or Suprefact(Hoechst) by daily subcutaneous injection
- Baseline endocrinology and ultrasound assessment to confirm downregulation
- Ovarian stimulation with Metrodin HP or Gonal F(Serono)
- Follicular phase monitoring after one week of stimulation

cycle day 19–21 start	baseline	monitoring
downregulation for 10–14 days	stimulation..8–12 days	36 hours......OCR......ET
Synarel or...............	...........FSH........................	hCG
Suprefact		Utrogestan or Cyclogest............

Baseline Assessment: Ultrasound

- Ovaries: Size, position
  Shape, texture
  Cysts
  Evidence of PCO
- Uterus: Endometrial size, shape, texture & thickness
  Fibroids
  Congenital or other anomalies/abnormalities
- Hydrosalpinges, loculated fluid

Baseline assessement: Endocrinology

- Oestradiol: less than 50 pg/ml
- LH: less than 5 IU/L.
- Progesterone: less than 2 ng/ml
  If any values are elevated:
    continue GnRH agonist treatment
    withold stimulation
    reassess 3–7 days later
- If LH remains elevated:
    withold stimulation
    increase dose of GnRH agonist
- (FSH: less than 10 IU/L without downregulation)

Ovarian stimulation

- Pure FSH by subcutaneous self-injection
- Starting dose:
  - according to age and/or history
    - age 35 or younger   150 IU/day
    - age over 35:   225 IU/day
  - depending on previous response,
    - up to 300–450 IU daily
- Begin monitoring after 7 days of stimulation
  (*adjusted according to history and baseline assessment*)

Cycle monitoring

Stimulation day 8 assessment

- Ultrasound assessment
  - Follicle size 14 mm or less: review in 2 or 3 days
  - Follicle size 16 mm or greater: review daily
- plasma oestradiol
- plasma LH
  - review as necessary

Induction of ovulation

- hCG 10 000 IU by subcutaneous injection when:
  - Leading follicle is at least 17–18 mm in diameter
  - 2 or more follicles >14 mm in diameter
  - Endometrium:
    - at least 8 mm in thickness with
    - trilaminar 'halo' appearance
  - Oestradiol levels approx.
    - 100–150 pg/ml per large follicle
- Oocyte retrieval scheduled for 34–36 hours post-hCG

gonadotrophin hormone (hCG) 5000–10 000 units (Profasi, Serono UK) when at least one leading follicle ≥ 18 mm diameter.

6. Oocyte retrieval is scheduled 34–36 hours after hCG injection, and luteal support per vaginum (PV) Utrogestan capsules, 100 mg three times daily (Besins-Iscovesco), Cyclogest pessaries 200 mg PV twice daily (Hoechst), or Gestone 50 mg daily by intramuscular injection (Ferring) is commenced on the day after hCG administration.
7. Oocyte retrieval is performed under vaginal ultrasound guidance, using disposable double-channelled needles (COOK IVF, K-OPSD 1632 XXET). Aspiration and follicle flushing are carried out using vacuum aspiration and infusion systems from COOK IVF (K-MAR Complete System).
  The aspirates are collected into heated 15 ml Falcon tubes.

Preparation for each case

The embryologist is involved in the management of each in vitro fertilization (IVF) case from the time that the treatment cycle is initiated, and there should be a system which ensures that all members of the laboratory staff can be familiar with the treatment plan for each patient. The laboratory staff should also ensure that all appropriate consent forms have been signed by both partners, including consent for special procedures and storage of cryopreserved embryos. Study all details of any previous assisted conception treatment, including response to stimulation, number and quality of oocytes, timing of insemination, fertilization rate, embryo quality, and embryo transfer procedure, and judge whether any parameters at any stage could be altered or improved in the present cycle. A repeat semen assessment may be required at the beginning of the treatment cycle, especially if the male partner has suffered recent illness, stress, or trauma which could affect spermatogenesis. If necessary, a back-up semen sample may also be cryopreserved after this assessment.

The risk of introducing any infection into the laboratory via gametes and samples must be absolutely minimized: note details of screening tests such as human immunodeficiency virus (HIV) and hepatitis B at the beginning of the treatment cycle, and repeat if necessary.

After administration of hCG to induce ovulation, the embryologist should again examine the case notes and prepare the laboratory records for the following day's oocyte retrievals, with attention to the following details:

1. Previous history, with attention to laboratory procedures: any modifications required?
2. Semen assessment: any special preparations or precautions required for sample collection or preparation?

3. Current cycle history: number of follicles, endocrine parameters, any suggestion of ovarian hyperstimulation syndrome?

Laboratory case notes, media, culture vessels and tubes for sperm preparation are prepared during the afternoon prior to each case, with clear and adequate labelling throughout. Tissue culture dishes or plates are equilibrated in the CO_2 incubator overnight.

The choice of culture system used is a matter of individual preference and previous experience; two systems which are both widely and successfully used by different IVF groups are described here :

Microdroplets under oil

Pour previously equilibrated mineral oil into 60 mm petri dishes which have been clearly marked with each patient's surname.

Using either a Pasteur pipette or adjustable pipettor and sterile tips, carefully place 8 or 9 droplets of medium around the edge of the dish. One or two drops may be placed centrally, to be used as wash drops.

Examination of the follicular growth records will indicate approximately how many drops/dishes should be prepared; each drop may contain one or two oocytes. Droplet size can range from 50 to 250 µl per drop.

Four-well plates

Prepare labelled and numbered plates containing 0.5–1 ml of tissue culture medium and equilibrate overnight in a humidified incubator. Each well is normally used to incubate three oocytes. Small petri dishes with approximately 2 ml of HEPES-containing medium may also be prepared, to be used for washing oocytes immediately after identification in the follicular aspirates. This system may also be used in combination with an overlay of equilibrated mineral oil, allowing the use of non-humidified incubators.

Oocyte retrieval (OCR) and identification

Before beginning each OCR procedure

1. Ensure that heating blocks, stages, and trays are warmed to 37 °C.
2. Pre-warm collection test tubes and 60 mm petri dishes for scanning aspirates.
3. Prepare a fire-polished Pasteur pipette + holder, a fine-drawn blunt Pasteur pipette as a probe for manipulations, and 1ml syringes with attached needles for dissection.
4. Check names on dishes and laboratory case notes with medical notes.

Examine follicular aspirates under a stereo dissecting microscope with transmitted illumination base and heated stage. Aliquot the contents of each test tube into two or three petri dishes, forming a thin layer of fluid which can be quickly, carefully, and easily scanned for the presence of an oocyte in the follicular tissue. Low power magnification (6–12 x) can be used for scanning the fluid, and oocyte identification verified using higher magnification (25–50 x).

The oocyte usually appears within varying quantities of cumulus cells and if very mature, may be pale and difficult to see (immature oocytes are dark and also difficult to see). Granulosa cells are clearer and more 'fluffy', present in amorphous, often iridescent clumps. Blood clots, especially from the collection needle, should be carefully dissected with 23g needles to check for the presence of cumulus cells.

When an oocyte/cumulus complex (OCC) is found, assess its stage of maturity by noting the volume, density, and condition of the surrounding coronal and cumulus cells. If the egg can be seen, the presence of a single polar body indicates that it has reached the stage of metaphase II.

There are reports relating the OCC appearance with maturity and fertilizing capacity of the oocyte, and the following scheme can be used for assessment:

1) *Germinal vesicle:* the oocyte is very immature. There is no expansion of the surrounding cells, which are tightly packed around the egg. A large nucleus (the germinal vesicle) is still present and may occasionally be seen with the help of an inverted microscope. Maturation occasionally takes place in vitro from this stage, and germinal vesicles are pre-incubated for 24 hours before insemination (Figure 10.1a).

2) *Metaphase I* (germinal vesicle breakdown, GVBD): the oocyte is surrounded by a tightly apposed layer of corona cells, and tightly packed cumulus may surround this with a maximum size of approximately five egg diameters. If the oocyte can be seen, it no longer shows a germinal vesicle. The absence of a polar body indicates that the oocyte is in metaphase I, and these immature eggs can be pre-incubated for 12–24 hours before insemination (Figure 10.1b).

3) *Metaphase II*
    (a) *Pre-ovulatory* (harvested from Graafian follicles): this is the optimal level of maturity, appropriate for successful fertilization. Coronal cells are still apposed to the egg, but are fully radiating; one polar body has been extruded. The cumulus has expanded into a fluffy mass (although beware the possibility that some may have been lost in aspiration) and can be easily stretched (Figure 10.1c).
    (b) *Very mature:* the egg can often be seen clearly as a pale orb; little coronal material is present and is dissociated from the egg. The cumulus is very profuse but is still cellular. The latest events of this stage involve a conden-

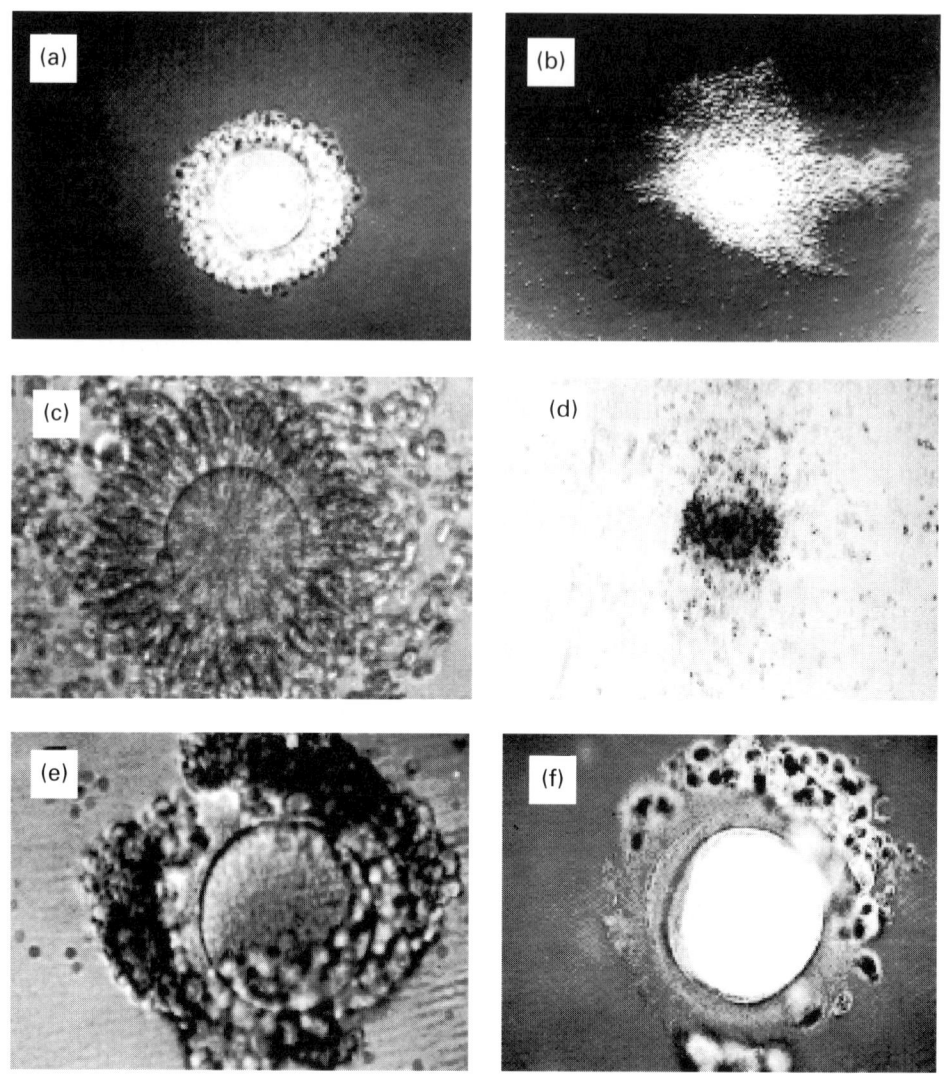

Figure 10.1 Phase contrast micrographs showing stages of human oocyte maturation normally encountered in ART. (a) germinal vesicle; (b) immature, metaphase I; (c) preovulatory, metaphase II; (d) post-mature; (e) luteinized; (f) atretic.

sation of cumulus into small black (refractile) drops, as if a tight corona is reforming around the egg (Figure 10.1d).
(c) *Luteinised:* the egg is very pale and often is difficult to find. The cumulus has broken down and becomes a gelatinous mass around the egg. These eggs have a low probability of fertilization, and are usually inseminated with little delay (Figure 10.1e).

(d) *Atretic:* granulosa cells are fragmented, and have a lace-like appearance. The oocyte is very dark, and can be difficult to identify (Figure 10.1f).

Gross morphological assessment of oocyte maturity is highly subjective, and subject to inaccuracies. Since 1990, micromanipulation procedures have been widely introduced into routine IVF; because the procedure involves completely denuding oocytes from surrounding cells using hyaluronidase, this allows accurate assessment of the cytoplasm and nuclear maturity. It is now apparent that gross OCC morphology does not necessarily correlate with nuclear maturity. Alikani *et al.* (1995) used intracytoplasmic sperm injection (ICSI) to analyse its developmental consequences in dysmorphic human oocytes. Of 2968 injected oocytes, 806 (27.2%) were classified as dysmorphic on the basis of cytoplasmic granularity, areas of necrosis, organelle clustering, vacuolation, or accumulating saccules of smooth endoplasmic reticulum. Anomalies of the zona pellucida and non-spherical oocytes were also noted.

No single abnormality was found to be associated with a reduction in fertilization rate, and fertilization was not compromised in oocytes with multiple abnormalities. Overall pregnancy and implantation rates were not altered in patients in whom at least one oocyte was dysmorphic; however, exclusive replacement of embryos which originated from dysmorphic oocytes led to a lower implantation rate, and a higher incidence of biochemical pregnancies. They suggest that aberrations in the morphology of oocytes, possibly a result of ovarian hyperstimulation, are of no consequence to fertilization or early cleavage after ICSI. It is possible that embryos generated from dysmorphic oocytes have a reduced potential for implantation and further development.

R. Homburg and M. Shelef (1995) have recently reviewed the factors affecting oocyte quality, including morphology, chromosome anomalies, age, follicular microenvironment (in relation to ovulation induction protocol), and endocrine factors. They concluded that nuclear maturity is an important factor in the assessment of oocyte quality, and that the environment of the oocyte has a significant effect upon its quality. LH plays a central role in the maturation process of the oocyte, and an imbalance in the secretion of LH may upset the mechanisms involved. LH is required for completion of the first meiotic division, and inappropriate secretion of LH impairs oocyte quality. A working hypothesis has been proposed which suggests that inappropriately high levels of LH cause a premature maturation of the oocyte, causing it to become physiologically aged, less readily fertilized, and, if embryo implantation occurs, it may be more prone to early abortion.

High follicular phase LH levels are a poor prognosis for IVF and pregnancy, and patients with a poor previous history of IVF, including poor oocyte and embryo quality, may benefit from management with long-term GnRH down-regulation and LH monitoring during the follicular phase.

> **Oocyte collection**
> 1 Scan follicular aspirates immediately, on a heated microscope stage
> 2 Wash oocytes, if necessary dissect free of blood clots or granulosa cells
> 3 Transfer immediately to culture system
> 4 At the end of the procedure, assess oocytes for quality and maturity, and record optimum time for insemination
> 5 For microdroplet/oil system, prepare oil dish(es) for insemination, and equilibrate in the incubator
> 6 Maintain stable pH and temperature throughout

Insemination

Oocytes are routinely inseminated with a concentration of 100 000 normal motile sperm per ml. If the prepared sperm shows suboptimal parameters of motility or morphology, the insemination concentration may be accordingly increased. Some reports have recently suggested that the use of a high insemination concentration (HIC) may be a useful prelude before deciding upon ICSI treatment for male factor patients.

Microdroplets under oil

At the end of the oocyte retrieval procedure, prepare insemination dishes by pouring mineral oil into the appropriate number of 60 mm petri dishes, and equilibrate these in the incubator along with the collected oocytes in their collection dishes.

Pre-ovulatory oocytes are inseminated after 3–4 hours pre-incubation in vitro. Each oocyte is transferred into a drop containing motile sperm at a concentration of approximately 100 000 per ml.

1. Assess the volume of sperm suspension required according to the number of oocytes, and make an appropriate dilution of prepared sperm in a test tube. Check the dilution by examining a drop of suspension on a plain glass slide under the microscope: it should contain 20 normal motile sperm per high power field (x 10). Adjust the dilution accordingly until the number of progressively motile normal sperm appears adequate.

2. Adjust the pH of the suspension by gently blowing 5% CO_2 over the surface, and incubate at 37 °C for 30 minutes.
3. Using a Pasteur pipette, place droplets of the sperm suspension into the paraffin dishes prepared at the end of the oocyte collection.
4. Examine each oocyte before transfer to the insemination drop; it may be necessary to dissect the cumulus in order to remove bubbles, large clumps of granulosa cells, or blood clots.
5. Prepare labelled 35 mm petri dishes containing equilibrated paraffin at this time. These will be used for culture of the zygotes after scoring for fertilisation the following day.

If the oocyte culture droplets have been created to a measured (eg. 240 μl) volume, the oocytes can be inseminated by adding 10 μl of prepared sperm suspension that has been adjusted to 2.5 million per ml (final concentration approximately 100 000 sperm per ml, or 25 000 per oocyte).

Four-well dishes

Add a measured volume of prepared sperm suspension to each well, to a total concentration of approximately 100 000 progressively motile sperm per well.

Scoring of fertilization on day 1

Embryo dissection

Inseminated oocytes must be dissected the day following insemination in order to assess fertilization. Oocytes at this time are normally covered with a layer of coronal and cumulus cells. These are carefully dissected away to clearly visualize the cell cytoplasm and examined for the presence of two pronuclei indicating normal fertilization. Scoring for pronuclei should be carried out between 17 and 20 hours after insemination, before pronuclei merge during syngamy. The choice of dissection procedure is a matter of individual preference, and sometimes a combination of methods may be necessary for particular cases. Whatever the method used, it must be carried out carefully, delicately, and speedily, taking care not to expose the fertilized eggs to changes in temperature and pH.

Dissection techniques

1. *Needle dissection:* use two 26g needles attached to 1ml syringes, microscope on 25x magnification. Use one needle as a guide, anchoring a piece of cellular

debris if possible; slide the other needle down the first one, 'shaving' cells from around the zona pellucida, with a scissors-like action.

2. *'Rolling':* use one 23g needle attached to a syringe, and a fine glass probe. With the microscope on 12x magnification, use the needle to score lines in each droplet on the base of the plastic dish. Adjust the magnification to 25x, and push the egg gently over the scratches with a fire polished glass probe until the adhering cells are teased away.

   Great care must be taken with either technique to avoid damaging the zona pellucida or the egg either by puncture or over-distortion. Breaks or cracks in the zona can sometimes be seen, and a small portion of the egg may extrude through the crack (this may have occurred during dissection or during the aspiration process). Occasionally, the zona is very fragile, fracturing or distorting at the slightest touch. In cases such as this, it is probably best not to continue the dissection. If no pronuclei have been seen, immediate re-insemination may be considered as a precaution.

3. *Narrow-gauge pipetting*

   Place the microscope on 25x magnification, and choose a drawn-out pipette with a diameter slightly larger than the egg. Attach a bulb to the pipette, and aspirate 2 cm of clean culture medium into it, providing a protective buffer. This allows easy flushing of the egg, and prevents it from sticking to the inside surface of the pipette.

   Place the pipette over the egg and gently aspirate it into the shaft.

   If the oocyte does not easily enter, change to a larger diameter pipette (however, if the diameter is too large, it will be ineffective for cumulus removal).

   Gently aspirate and expel the egg through the pipette, retaining the initial buffer volume, until sufficient cumulus and corona is removed, allowing clear visualization of the cell cytoplasm and pronuclei.

Making narrow gauge pipettes

The preparation of finely-drawn pipettes with an inner diameter slightly larger than the circumference of an egg is an acquired skill which requires practice and patience. Hold both ends of the pipette, and roll an area approximately 2.5 cm below the tapered section of the pipette over a gentle flame (bunsen or spirit burner). As the glass begins to melt, quickly pull the pipette in both directions to separate, and carefully and quickly (before the glass has a chance to cool) break the pipette at an appropriate position. It is important that the tip should have a clean break, without rough or uneven edges; these will damage the egg during dissection. Always examine the tip of each pipette to ensure that it is of accurate diameter, with smooth clean edges. (Commercially prepared fine-drawn pipettes have recently become available, from COOK IVF and SWEMED).

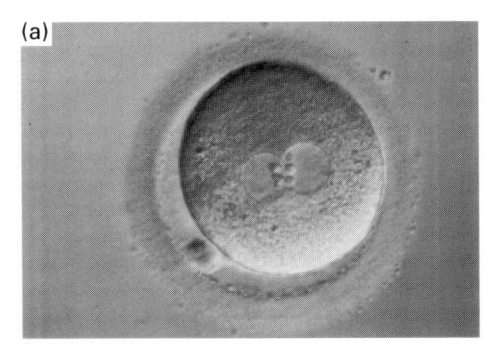

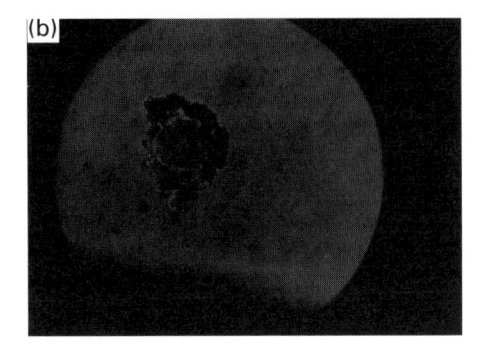

Figure 10.2 Phase contrast micrographs of fertilized human eggs. (a) Two pronuclei, normal fertilization; (b) three pronuclei, abnormal fertilization.

Scoring of pronuclei

An inverted microscope is recommended for accurate scoring of fertilization; although the pronuclei can be seen with dissecting microscopes, it can often be difficult to distinguish normal pronuclei from vacuoles or other irregularities in the cytoplasm. Normally fertilized eggs should have two pronuclei, two polar bodies, regular shape with intact zona pellucida, and a clear healthy cytoplasm. A variety of different features may be observed: the cytoplasm of normally fertilized eggs is usually slightly granular, whereas the cytoplasm of unfertilized eggs tends to be completely clear and featureless. The cytoplasm can vary from slightly granular and healthy-looking, to brown or dark and degenerate. The shape of the egg may also vary, from perfectly spherical to irregular (Figure 10.2).

Single pronucleate zygotes obtained after conventional IVF have recently been analysed by fluorescent in situ hybridization (FISH) to determine their ploidy: of 16 zygotes, 10 were haploid and six were diploid (4 XY and 2 XX) It seems that during the course of their interaction, it is possible for human gamete nuclei to associate together and form diploid, single pronucleate zygotes. These findings confirm a newly recognized variation of human pronuclear interaction during syngamy, and the authors suggest that single pronucleate zygotes which develop with normal cleavage may be safely replaced (Levron *et al.* 1995).

Details of morphology and fertilization should be recorded for each zygote, for reference when choosing embryos for transfer on day 2.

Remove zygotes with normal fertilization at the time of scoring from the insemination drops or wells, transfer into new dishes or plates containing pre-equilibrated culture medium, and return them to the incubator for a further 24 hours of culture. Those with abnormal fertilization such as multipronucleate zygotes, must be cultured separately, so that there is no possibility of their being selected for embryo transfer; after cleavage these are indistinguishable from normally fertilized oocytes.

Although the presence of two pronuclei confirms fertilization, their absence does not necessarily indicate fertilization failure, and may instead represent either parthenogenetic activation, or a delay in timing of one or more of the events involved in fertilization. A study has shown that in 40% of oocytes with no sign of fertilization 17–27 hours after insemination, 41% had the appearance of morphologically normal embryos on the following day, with morphology and cleavage rate similar to that of eggs with obvious pronuclei on day 1. However, 30% of these zygotes arrested on day 2, compared with only 7% of 'normally' fertilized oocytes (Plachot *et al.* 1993), and they showed a reduced implantation rate of 6% compared with 11.1%. Cytogenetic analysis of these embryos revealed a higher incidence of chromosomal anomalies (55% versus 29%), and a high rate of haploidy (20%), confirming parthenogenetic activation. Nine per cent were triploid, and 26% mosaic (Plachot *et al.* 1988).

Delayed fertilization with the appearance of pronuclei on day 2 may also be observed, and these embryos tend to have an impaired developmental potential. Oehninger *et al.* (1989) suggest that delayed fertilization can be attributed to morphological or endocrine oocyte defects in 37% of their cases, and sperm defects in 14.8%. Thirty-three per cent of the cases studied had no obvious association with either oocyte or sperm defects.

Re-insemination

Although oocytes which fail to demonstrate clear pronuclei at the time of scoring for fertilization can be re-inseminated, this practice has been widely questioned scientifically. Fertilization or cleavage may then be seen on day 2, but this may be as a consequence of the initial insemination, and the delay in fertilization may be attributed either to functional disorders of the sperm, or maturation delay of the oocyte. These embryos generally have a poor prognosis for implantation; however, complete failure of fertilization on day 1 is a devastating crisis for the couple, and extremely difficult for them to accept without further attempted action. As everyone who has experience of IVF will testify, even the most unlikely and improbable circumstances can sometimes result in the birth of a healthy baby.

The re-insemination procedure should be carried out as early as possible. If the husband is not available to produce a second sample within 26–28 hours of the oocyte retrieval, the original insemination sample should be re-examined for motility and used at least as an interim measure.

Selection of surplus pronucleate embryos for cryopreservation

If a large number of oocytes have two clearly visible pronuclei on day 1, a selected number can be kept in culture for transfer on day 2, and the remainder considered for pronucleate stage cryopreservation. The decision as to the number of embryos to be frozen at the pronucleate stage should take into consideration the patient's previous history regarding cleavage and quality of embryos. Embryos to be frozen should have a regular outline, distinct zona, and clearly visible pronuclei. The cryopreservation procedure must be initiated while the pronuclei are still visible, before the onset of syngamy.

Embryo quality and selection for transfer

On day 2 (approximately 48–54 hours after oocyte retrieval), oocytes with normal fertilization and cleavage may contain from two to eight blastomeres. The embryos should then be carefully evaluated to select those with the highest implantation potential. The limitations of evaluating embryos based on morphological criteria alone are well recognised: correlations between gross morphology and implantation are weak and inaccurate, unless the embryos are clearly fragmenting. Many studies have researched more objective criteria for judging embryo viability and implantation potential, including delayed embryo transfer with culture to blastocyst stage, measurement of metabolic activity and secretions by assaying culture medium, and embryo biopsy followed by pre-implantation genetic diagnosis.

These methods are excellent tools for research in specialized laboratories, and may eventually lead to the development of accurate embryo assessment. It is also possible that in the future the techniques will be simplified and refined to the extent that they may be more widely accessible and available. At the moment it is difficult to incorporate these selection procedures into a routine IVF practice, and we are left with subjective morphological assessment, which, although unsatisfactory, is quick, non-invasive, and easy to carry out in routine practice.

Standard morphological criteria used in evaluating embryo quality include the rate of division judged by the number of blastomeres, size, shape, symmetry, and cytoplasmic appearance of the blastomeres, and the presence of anucleate cytoplasmic fragments.

Based upon these critera, embryos may be thus arbitrarily classified:

Grade 1

Embryos have even, regular, spherical blastomeres with moderate refractility (i.e. not very dark) and with intact zona. Allowance must be made for the appearance of blastomeres that are in division or that have divided asynchronously with their sisters, e.g. 3, 5, 6, or 7 cell embryos. These may be uneven but are perfectly normal. As always, individual judgement is important, and this is a highly subjective assessment. Grade 1 embryos have no, or very few, fragments (less than 10%) (Figure 10.3a).

Grade 2

Embryos have uneven or irregularly shaped blastomeres, with mild variation in refractility and no more than 10% fragmentation of blastomeres (Figure 10.3b).

Grade 3

Embryos show fragmentation of no more than 50% of blastomeres. The remaining blastomeres must be at least in reasonable (Grade 2) condition and with refractility associated with cell viability; the zona pellucida must be intact (Figure 10.3c).

Grade 4

More than 50% of the blastomeres are fragmented, and there may be gross variation in refractility. Remaining blastomeres should appear viable (Figure 10.3d).

Grade 5

Zygotes with two pronuclei on day 2, either as a result of delayed fertilization or reinsemination on day 1.

Grade 6

Embryos are non-viable, with lysed, contracted, or dark blastomeres.

In an attempt to more clearly define morphological criteria that might be used for embryo assessment, Cohen *et al.* carried out a detailed analysis using videocinematography (1989). Immediately before embryo transfer, embryos were recorded on VHS for 30–90 seconds, at several focal points, using Nomarski optics and an overall magnification of 1400x. The recordings were subsequently analysed by observers who were unaware of the outcome of the IVF procedure, and they objectively assessed a total of 11 different parameters:

Cell organelles visible	Cellular extrusions
Blastomeres all intact	Cytoplasmic vacuoles
Identical blastomere size	Blastomeres contracted
Smooth membranes	
Dark blastomeres	% variation in zona thickness
Cell–cell adherence	% extracellular fragments

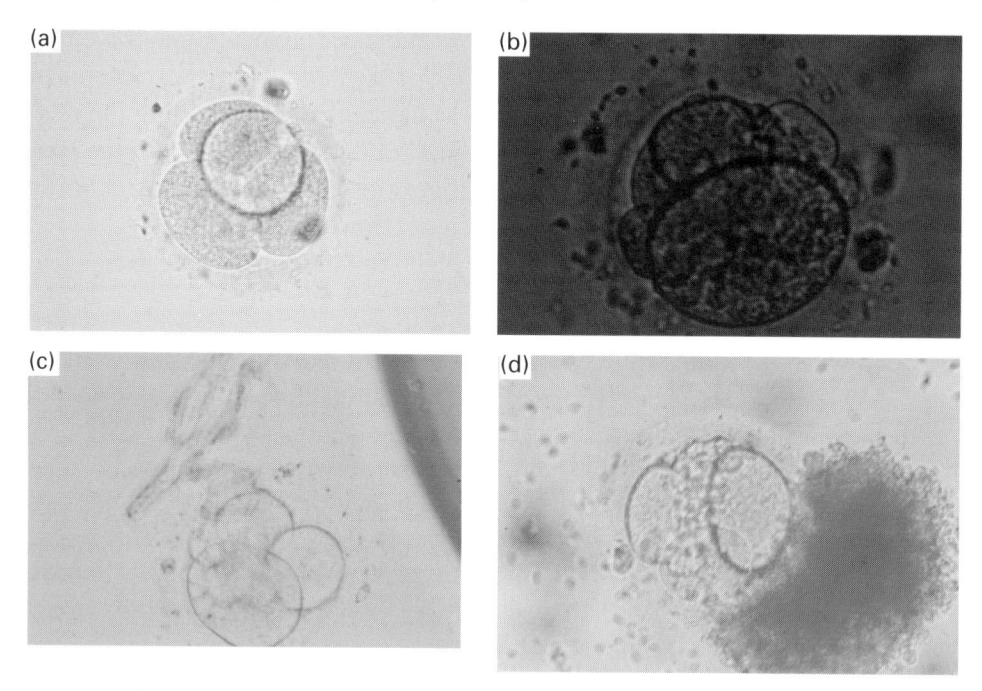

Figure 10.3 Photographs of morphological variations in human embryos 2 days after fertilization in vitro. (a) Four regular blastomeres, no fragments; (b) uneven blastomeres, approximately 10% fragmentation; (c) three blastomeres approximately 20% fragmentation; (d) two blastomeres, approximately 50% fragmentation.

Nine parameters were judged (+) or (−), and variation in zona thickness and percentage of extracellular fragments were given a numerical value. Analysis of these criteria showed that the most important predictor of fresh embryo implantation was the percentage of variation in thickness of the zona pellucida. Embryos with a thick, even zona had a poor prognosis for implantation; those whose zona had thin patches also had 'swollen', more refractile blastomeres, and had few or no fragments.

In analysing frozen-thawed embryos, the best predictor of implantation was cell–cell adherence. The proportion of thawed embryos with more than one abnormality (77%) was higher than that of fresh embryos (38%) despite similar implantation rates (18% versus 15%)

Fragments

Most IVF embryologists would agree that fragmentation is the norm in routine IVF, but it is not clear whether this is an effect of culture conditions and follicular stimulation, or a characteristic of human development. The degree of fragmentation varies from 5 or 10% to 100%, and the fragments may be either localized or scattered. Alikani & Cohen (1995) used an analysis of patterns of cell fragmentation in the human embryo as a means of determining the relationship between cell fragmentation and implantation potential, with the conclusion that not only the degree, but also the pattern of embryo fragmentation determine its implantation potential.

Five distinct patterns of fragmentation which can be seen by day 3 were identified:

1. <5% of the volume of the perivitelline space occupied by fragments
2. All or most fragments localized, concentrated in one area of the perivitelline space, with five or more normal cells visible.
3. Fragments scattered throughout, and similar in size
4. Large fragments, indistinguishable from blastomeres, and scattered throughout the perivitelline space (PVS); usually associated with very few cells.
5. Fragments throughout the PVS, appearing degenerate such that cell boundaries are invisible, associated with contracted and granular cytoplasm.

Implantation potential was greatest in types 1 and 2, and diminished in types 3 and 4. In 15 years of clinical embryology, there are no definitive reports on the causes of fragmentation, although speculations include high spermatozoal numbers and consequently high levels of free radicals, temperature or pH shock, and stimulation protocols. Observed through the scanning electron microscope, the surface of fragments is made up of irregularly shaped blebs and protrusions, very different to the regular surface of blastomeres, which is organised into short, regular microvilli (Figure 10.4). Interestingly, programmed cell death in somatic cells also starts with surface blebbing, and is caused, in part, by a calcium-induced disorganization of the cytoskeleton. We can speculate that similar mechanisms operate within human embryos, but we have so far no scientific evidence that this is the case. There does appear to be an element of programming in this partial embryonic autodestruction, as embryos from certain patients, irrespective of the types of procedure applied in successive IVF attempts, are always prone to fragmentation. Fragments may be removed during micromanipulation for assisted hatching, and there is growing evidence that fragment removal may improve implantation. Surprisingly, fragmented embryos, repaired or not, do implant and often come to term. This demonstrates the highly regulative nature of the human embryo, as it can apparently lose over half of its cellular mass and still recover, and also confirms the general consensus that the mature oocyte contains much more material than it needs for development. The reasons why part, and only part, of an early embryo should become disorganized and degenerate are a mystery. Different

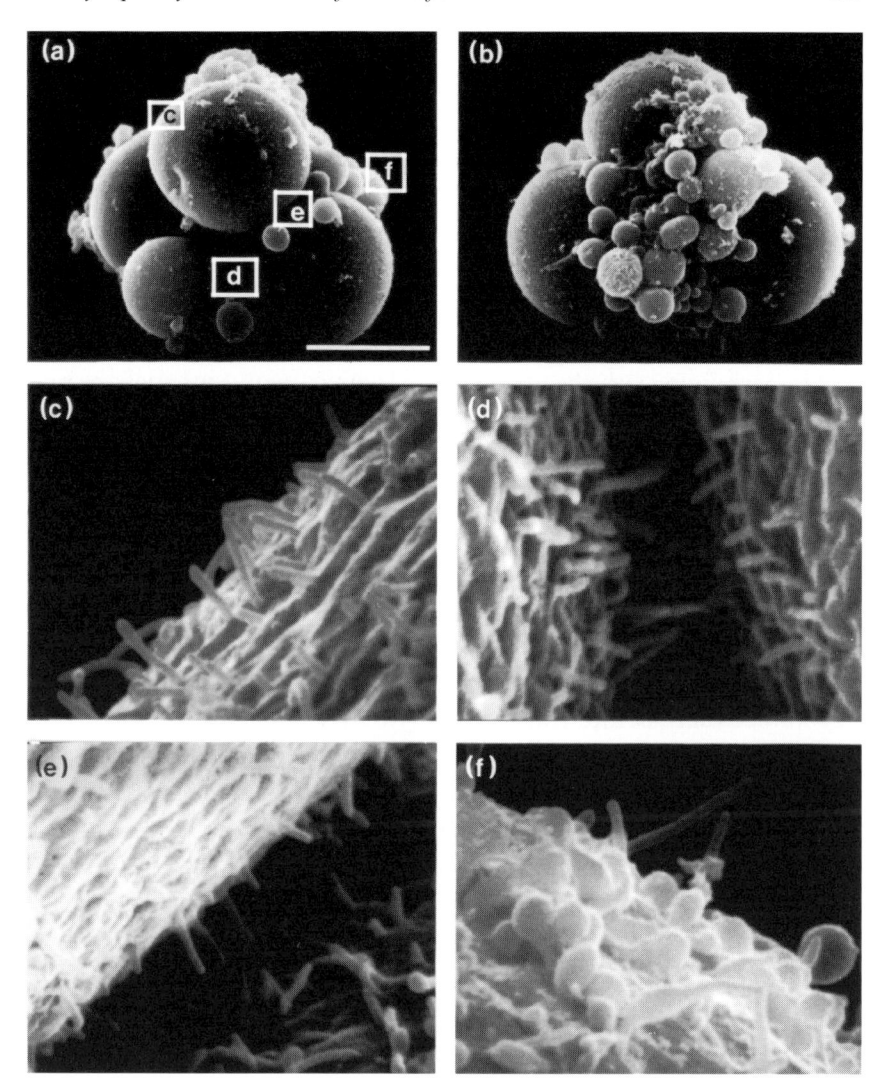

Figure 10.4 Scanning electron micrographs. (a, b) Two views of a human four-cell embryo showing 20% fragmentation (c–e) magnification of corresponding areas showing regular short microvilli of vital blastomeres and intercellular areas; (f) magnification of the surface of a cytoplasmic fragment showing irregular blebs and protrusions.

degrees of fragmentation argue against the idea that the embryo is purposely casting off excess cytoplasm, somewhat analogous to the situation in annelids and marsupials that shed cytoplasmic lobes rich in yolk, and favours the idea of partial degeneration. Perhaps it involves cell polarization, where organelles gather to one side of the cell. It is certain that pH, calcium, and transcellular currents trigger cell polarisation, which may in certain cases lead to an abnormal polarization, and therefore to fragmentation. These areas are for the moment wide open to speculation, and studies are in progress.

Embryo transfer

Historically, routine embryo transfer has been carried out on day 2, approximately 48 hours after oocyte retrieval. Delaying embryo transfer until day 3 has shown no detrimental effects on pregnancy rates, and may be of benefit in selecting embryos with a better prognosis for development. Recently, co-culture techniques have been introduced which greatly enhance the rate of blastocyst formation in vitro, and it has now been suggested that day 5 transfer of blastocysts rather than earlier transfer of cleavage stage embryos will significantly enhance implantation.

When selecting the 'best' quality embryos for transfer, we must appreciate that the time during which this observation and judgment is made represents only a tiny instant of a rapidly evolving process of development. Embryos can be judged quite differently at two different periods in time, as may be seen if a comparison is made between assessments made in the morning, and later in the day immediately before transfer. Individual judgment should be exercised in determining which embryos are selected. In general, those embryos at later stages and of higher grades are preferred, but the choice is often not clear cut. The Grade 2 category covers a wide range of morphological states but, provided the blastomeres are not grossly abnormal, a later stage Grade 2 embryo may be selected in preference to an earlier stage Grade 1 embryo. Attention should also be paid to the appearance of the zona pellucida and to the pattern of fragmentation. Embryos of Grade 3 or 4 are transferred only where no better embryos are available. If only pronucleate embryos are available on day 2, they should be cultured further and transferred only if cleavage occurs.

The recent application of pre-implantation genetic diagnosis by FISH analysis of biopsied blastomeres has shown a surprising discrepancy between gross morphology and genetic normality of the embryos, in that even the most 'beautiful' embryos may have genetic abnormalities, whilst those with less aesthetic qualities, including the presence of fragments, may in fact have normal implantation potential.

Remaining embryos

Embryos of Grade 1 or 2 which remain after the embryo transfer procedure may be cryopreserved. Remaining cleaved embryos unsuitable for freezing can be kept in culture and scored daily until day 6. Those which develop to blastocyst stage on day 5 or day 6 can also be cryopreserved.

Embryo transfer procedure

Materials

1. Pre-equilibrated, warmed culture medium.
2. 1 ml disposable syringe
3. Embryo transfer catheter
4. Sterile disposable gloves (non-powdered)
5. Clean petri dish
6. Fire-polished Pasteur pipette and glass probe
7. Dissecting microscope with warm stage

Although it may seem obvious that correct identification of patient and embryos is vital, errors in communication do happen and can lead to a disastrous mistake, especially should there be patients with similar names undergoing treatment at the same time. Therefore, a routine discipline of identification should be followed to avoid any possibility of a mistake:

1. Ensure that medical notes always accompany a patient who is being prepared for embryo transfer.
2. Name and medical numbers on medical notes and patient identity bracelet should be checked by two people, i.e. the clinician in charge of the procedure and the assisting nurse.
3. The doctor should also check name and number verbally with the patient, and doctor, nurse, and patient may sign an appropriate form confirming that the details are correct.
4. The duty embryologist should check the same details with the embryology records, and also sign the same form in the presence of the doctor.

Preparation of embryos for transfer

Legislation in the UK now prohibits the transfer of more than three embryos in a treatment cycle, and the transfer of two embryos is recommended for patients with a good prognosis (i.e. young age, tubal infertility only, previous history of pregnancy and/or delivery).

1. When the embryos for transfer have been identified, scored, and their details recorded, place those that are to be transferred together in fresh medium in a single droplet under oil, or in a single well. No more than three embryos should be transferred.
2. After gently pushing the embryos together, leave them under low power on the heated stage of the microscope, in focus.
3. Turn off the microscope light.
4. Wash your hands with a surgical scrub preparation, and don sterile gloves.
5. Fill a 1 ml sterile syringe with warm medium, and eject any air bubbles.

6. Check that the catheter to be used moves freely though its outer sheath, attach it to the syringe, and eject the medium from the syringe through the catheter, discarding the medium.
7. Draw up warm medium through the catheter into the syringe, and then push the piston down to the 10 µl mark, ejecting excess medium and again discarding it.
8. Pour some clean warm medium into the warm petri dish on the microscope stage (for rinsing the catheter tip).
9. Place the end of the catheter carefully into the drop or well, away from the embryos, and inject a small amount of medium to break the boundary of surface tension that may appear at the end of the catheter. Aspirate the embryos into the catheter, so that the volume to be transferred is 15–20 µl.
10. If the embryos have been loaded from a droplet under oil, rinse the tip of the catheter in the petri dish containing clean warm medium.

Hand the catheter and syringe to the clinician for transfer to the patient. When the catheter is returned after the procedure, carefully inspect it, rotating under the microscope. It is especially important to ensure that no embryo is buried in any mucus present; note and record the presence of mucus and/or blood. Loosen the lueur fitting, and allow the fluid in the catheter to drain into the clean petri dish while continuing to observe through the microscope. Inform the doctor and patient as soon as you have confirmed that no embryos have been returned. If any embryos have been returned, they should be re-loaded into a clean catheter, and the transfer procedure repeated. If difficulties arise during the transfer procedure causing delay, return the embryos to the culture drop in the interim, until the physician is confident that they can be safely transferred to the uterus of the patient.

Gamete intrafallopian transfer (GIFT)

The World Collaborative Report on Assisted Reproduction published in 1993 summarized the results of 99 314 IVF transfer cycles, with a clinical pregnancy rate of 17.9% and live birth rate of 12.9%. Although GIFT represented only 10% of the total number of cycles compared with IVF, the clinical pregnancy rate for this procedure was 29.3%, with a live birth rate of 20.8%. Discussion continues as to the relative merits of intrauterine versus intratubal transfer, but it may be that intratubal transfer of gametes does have advantages: embryo development in a beneficial tubal microenvironment avoids the possible hazards of in vitro culture, especially if optimal laboratory conditions are not available. In addition, the embryo undergoes physiological passage into the uterus for implantation, avoiding endometrial trauma, and there is a diminished possibility of

---

Luteal phase support

- Utrogestan capsules (Besins-Iscovesco)
    100 mg tds or 200 mg tds pv
- or Cyclogest pessaries (Hoechst)
    200 mg bd or 400 mg bd pv
- or Gestone (Ferring)
    50 mg or 100 mg daily by im injection

Luteal phase support continues until day 77 post OCR, then is gradually withdrawn

---

embryo expulsion from the uterus immediately after transfer. The gametes may be transferred to the fallopian tubes via the fimbrial end, under laparoscopic guidance, or intracervically under ultrasound-guided control. In either case, the dynamics of the injection procedure are critical, and gametes should be transferred in less than 50 µl of fluid, at a very slow injection rate of 1 µl per second. The catheter must of course be precisely located using ultrasound guidance for transcervical procedures.

Gift procedure

1. Obtain the semen sample at least 2 hours prior to the start of the procedure, and prepare as for IVF to a final concentration of 3–5 million motile sperm per ml (so that 100 000–200 000 sperm are transferred to the fallopian tube).
2. Warm the sperm preparation, medium, and 2 × 35 mm petri dishes at 37 °C.
3. At the end of the oocyte retrieval procedure, select good quality mature eggs for transfer, and wash them in a small amount of medium in a warmed dish or test tube.
4. Place a droplet (50–100 µl) of sperm suspension in a warmed petri dish, and transfer the selected washed oocytes into this droplet.
5. Rinse a 0.5 ml Hamilton syringe and GIFT catheter with warm medium, and then load the catheter:
    i) 20 µl air
    ii) 30–40 µl oocytes + sperm
    iii) 10–20 µl air
6. Transfer the oocytes and sperm to the fallopian tube with minimum delay, to prevent exposing them to temperature fluctuations.
7. After transfer, expel medium remaining in the catheter and examine the droplet and the catheter carefully to ensure that no oocytes have been returned.

If there is an insufficient volume of adequately prepared sperm, the sperm and oocytes can be loaded separately:

 i) 20 µl air
 ii) 10–15 µl sperm
 iii) 10 µl oocytes in culture medium
 iv) 10–15 µl sperm
 v) 20 µl air

This method is also preferred by some couples for religious or philosophical reasons, as it theoretically avoids in vitro mixing of the gametes – oocytes and sperm come into contact after being expelled into the fallopian tube, where the process of fertiization may occur as in natural conception.

8. Surplus oocytes remaining after the GIFT procedure may be cultured for IVF – in cases of male infertility, confirmation that fertilization may take place is a useful diagnostic test. Resulting embryos can be cryopreserved if they fulfill the required criteria for cryopreservation.

Transport IVF

The facilities of a central expert IVF laboratory can be used to offer treatment in hospitals which do not have the necessary laboratory space and personnel. Carefully selected patients undergo ovarian stimulation, monitoring, and oocyte retrieval under the care and management of a gynaecologist who has a close liasion with an IVF laboratory team in a location which can be reached within 2 hours of the hospital or clinic where the oocyte retrieval procedure takes place. It is essential that only patients with simple, uncomplicated infertility and good ovarian response are selected, and that there should be very close communication and coordination between the patient, physician, and IVF laboratory team. The successful system of transport IVF at the Royal Liverpool University Hospital in the UK (C.R. Kingsland and M.M. Biljan, personal communication) recommend that strict patient inclusion criteria should be adhered to, as follows:

1. Women 35 years of age or less
2. Tubal damage as the sole cause of subfertility
3. Two normal recent semen analyses

Patients who do not satisfy these criteria should be referred for specialised treatment in the Central Unit.

Exclusion criteria:

1. Women over 35 years of age
2. Patients with LH:FSH ratio higher than 3:1
3. Patients with laparoscopically proven moderate or severe endometriosis
4. Male factor infertility

5. Patients requesting oocyte donation or donor insemination
6. Three previously unsuccessful IVF treatment cycles

A GnRH-agonist/FSH long protocol is used for superovulation so that a simplified monitoring regimen can be used (ultrasound assessment and optional serum oestradiol levels) and to allow scheduled admission of patients into the stimulation phase. This protocol also allows latitude in the administration of hCG, so that the timing of oocyte retrieval can be scheduled in a routine operating list. Profasi (hCG) 5000 IU is administered 36 hours prior to the planned follicular aspiration.

The couple under treatment must visit the central unit before hCG is given, both to receive detailed information and consent forms, and to familiarize themselves with the journey and the facilities. The husband will return to the central unit on the morning of oocyte retrieval to produce a semen sample and to collect a pre-warmed portable incubator. The portable incubator, plugged into a car cigarette lighter, is then used to transport the follicular aspirates which have been collected in the peripheral hospital or clinic. Follicular aspirates are collected under ultrasound-guided control into sterile test tubes (without flushing). It is essential that each test tube is *filled completely* and tightly capped in order to prevent pH fluctuations. A heated test tube rack during aspiration must be used to prevent temperature fluctuations in the aspirates. The presence of blood in the aspirates has not been found to adversely affect the outcome of fertilization, embryo development, and success rates. At the end of the oocyte retrieval procedure, the partner transports the follicular aspirates, together with the treatment records, to the central laboratory for oocyte identification and subsequent insemination and culture.

The embryo transfer procedure is carried out 48 hours later at the central unit. Patient follow-up is carried out by the physician at the peripheral unit.

Provided that the instructions and inclusion criteria are strictly adhered to, a highly motivated, well coordinated team working in close liaison can achieve success rates comparable to those obtained in the specialist centre, and IVF treatment can thus be offered to couples to whom it might otherwise be unavailable.

Coculture systems

Homologous and autologous co-culture systems which culture embryos in the presence of a layer of 'feeder' cells have been used to improve embryo development in vitro, and to try to overcome the phenomenon of developmental arrest which commonly occurs in routine in vitro culture. For the same developmental stage, cocultured embryos have higher numbers of cells and a fully cohesive inner cell mass when compared with embryos cultured in simple media It is postulated that improved development occurs as a result of four different possible mechanisms:

1. 'Metabolic locks': coculture cell layers can provide a supply of small molecular weight metabolites which simpler culture media lack. This supply may assist continued cell metabolism required for genome activation, and divert the potential for abnormal metabolic processes which may lead to cleavage arrest.
2. Growth factors essential for development may be supplied by the feeder cell layer.
3. Toxic compounds resulting from cell metabolism can be removed: heavy metal ions may be chelated by glycine produced by feeder cells, and ammonium and urea may be recycled through feeder cell metabolic cycles.
4. Feeder cells can synthesize reducing agents which prevent the formation of free radicals.

Coculture systems used include foetal calf endometrial fibroblasts, human ampullary and endometrial cell lines, granulosa cells, and a commercially produced cell line of Vero (African Green Monkey Kidney) cells. Before making the decision to use coculture as a clinical tool in IVF, the disadvantages of the system must be carefully considered:

1. The establishment of cell monolayers is laborious and time consuming; explants must be subcultured, with the establishment of appropriate culture conditions; cell morphology and growth patterns change with length of time and number of passages in culture.
2. Feeder cell medium is very rapidly metabolized, and medium pH can rapidly change to a level which embryos will not tolerate.
3. Reproducible conditions can be difficult to maintain.
4. Cell layers are very susceptible to bacterial, viral, and mycoplasmal contamination. Screening is essential: there is a risk of disease transmission to the embryo, and both cells and medium must be rigorously checked for viruses, bacteria, fungi, and mycoplasma.

Vero cell lines, used in vaccine preparation, are commercially available from the WHO library: reference Vero 6758, at passage 134, non-hazardous to human (Public Health Laboratory Service, European Collection of Animal Cell Culture, Salisbury, UK). These cells are not tumorigenic before passage 162, contain no extraneous viruses, and can be used to very carefully set up and maintain a well-organized coculture system. Frozen cells are thawed and seeded in culture flasks at 2–3 million cells per flask. Confluence is reached within 4 days, normally at a cell density of 6–8 million cells per flask. These first passage flasks are subcultured after trypsinisation into three samples:

1. Freeze one sample for future use, as cells must not be repeatedly passaged from flasks.
2. Seed a new flask.
3. Seed culture wells at a density of 100 000 cells per well – these wells reach confluence within three days.

> Note: Do not trypsinize cells more than seven times
> Do not use them after passage 142
> After four subcultures, screen the cells for chlamydia and mycoplasma (BioMérieux Kits 5532/1 and 4240/2)

Wells seeded on a Friday can be used during the whole of the following week, and are rinsed only once. Each patient has her own plates, regardless of the number of embryos to be cocultured, and plates are discarded immediately after use. Wells must never be re-used for different patients. The wells are rinsed with fresh medium 1 hour before adding embryos, which may be cocultured either at the pronucleate zygote stage on day 1, or at an early cleavage stage on day 2. Using this culture system, Menezo *et al.* (1995) improved their blastocyst development rate from 20% without coculture to 48–60%, and obtained an overall pregnancy rate per transfer of 42%, with an implantation rate per blastocyst of 20%.

Trypsinization

1. Wash monolayer with 5 ml Hank's balanced salt solution
2. Add 1.5 ml of 0.25% Trypsin + 0.2% EDTA in Ca/Mg free phosphate buffered saline
3. Incubate for 5 mins at 37 °C.
4. Add 5 ml culture medium + 5% serum and resuspend cells.
5. Centrifuge, 800 g 10 minutes.
6. Resuspend cells in 5 ml culture medium and count with a haemocytometer
7. Seed 4–well dishes at a seeding density of 100 000 cells/well, in 1ml of medium.
8. Incubate for 3 days before using for coculture.

Further reading

Alikani, M., & Cohen J. (1995) Patterns of cell fragmentation in the human embryo in vitro. *Journal of Assisted Reproduction and Genetics* **12** (Suppl.): 28s.

Alikani, M., Palermo, G., Adler, A., Bertoli, M., Blake, M. & Cohen, J. (1995) Intracytoplasmic sperm injection in dysmorphic human oocytes. *Zygote* **3**: 283–288.

Almeida, P.A. & Bolton, V.N. (1993) Immaturity and chromosomal abnormalities in oocytes that fail to develop pronuclei following insemination in vitro. *Human Reproduction* **8**: 229–232.

Almeida, P.A. & Bolton, V.N. (1995) The effect of temperature fluctuations on the cytoskeletal organisation and chromosomal constitution of the human oocyte. *Zygote* **3**: 357–365.

Angell, R.R., Templeton, A.A. & Aitken, R.J. (1986) Chromosome studies in human in vitro fertilization. *Human Genetics* **72**: 333.

Asch, R.H,. Balmaceda, J.P., Ellsworth, L.R. & Wong, P.C. (1985) Gamete Intrafallopian Transfer (GIFT): a new treatment for infertility. *International Journal of Fertility* **30**: 41.

Ashwood-Smith, M.J., Hollands, P. & Edwards R.G. (1989) The use of Albuminar (TM) as a medium supplement in clinical IVF. *Human Reproduction* **4**: 702–705.

Belaisch-Allart, J. (1991) Delayed embryo transfer in an in-vitro fertilization programme: how to avoid working on Sunday. *Human Reproduction* **6**: 541–543.

Bolton, V.N. (1991) Pregnancies after in vitro fertilization and transfer of human blastocysts. *Fertility and Stertility* **55**: 830–832.

Bolton, V.N., Hawes, S.M., Taylor, C.T. & Parsons, J.H. (1989) Development of spare human preimplantation embryos in vitro: an analysis of the correlations among gross morphology, cleavage rates, and development to the blastocyst. *Journal of In Vitro Fertilization and Embryo Transfer* **7**: 186.

Bongso, A., Ng, S.C. & Ratnam, S. (1990) Coculture: their relevance to assisted reproduction. *Human Reproduction* **5**: 893–900.

Brinsden, P.R. ((1994) Clinical experience with highly purified FSH. *Newsletter: Gonadotrophin for the 90s*, vol. 1 no.1, Excerpta Medica Asia Ltd.

Caro, C. & Trounson, A. (1986) Successful fertilization and embryo development, and pregnancy in human in vitro fertilization (IVF) using a chemically defined culture medium containing no protein. *Journal of In Vitro Fertilization and Embryo Transfer* **3**: 215–217.

Cohen, J. (1991) Assisted hatching of human embryos. *Journal of In Vitro Fertilization* and Embryo Transfer **8**: 179–189.

Cohen, J., Alikani, M., Trowbridge, J. & Rosenwaks, Z. (1992) Implantation enhancement by selective assisted hatching using zona drilling of embryos with poor prognosis. *Human Reproduction* **7**: 685–691.

Cohen, J., Inge, K.L., Suzman, M., Wiker, S.R. & Wright, G. (1989) Video-cinematography of fresh and cryopreserved embryos: a retrospective analysis of embryonic morphology and implantation. *Fertility and Sterility* **51**: 820.

Critchlow, J.D. (1989) Quality control in an in-vitro fertilization laboratory: use of human sperm survival studies *Human Reproduction* **4**: 545–549.

Danforth, R.A., Piana, S.D. & Smith, M. (1987). High purity water: an important component for success in in vitro fertilization. *American Biotechnology Laboratory* **5**: 58–60.

Edwards, R.G. & Purdy, J.M. (1982) *Human Conception In Vitro* Academic Press, London, New York.

Fishel, S. & Symonds, E.M. (1986) *IVF – Past, Present, and Future.* IRL Press, Oxford, Washington DC.

Gott, A.L., Hardy, K., Winston, R.M.L. & Leese, H.J. (1990) Noninvasive measurement of pyruvate and glucose uptake and lactate production by single human preimplantation embryos. *Human Reproduction* **5**: 104–110.

Grifo, J.A., Boyle, A. & Fischer, E. (1990) Preembryo biopsy and analysis of blastomeres by in situ hybridisation. *American Journal of Obstetrics and Gynecology* **163**: 2013–2019.

Hammitt, D.G., Walker, D.L. & Syrop, C.H. (1990).Improved methods for preparation of culture media for in-vitro fertilization and gamete intra-fallopian transfer *Human Reproduction* **5**: 457–463.

Handyside, A.H., Kontogianni, E.H., Hardy, K. & Winston R.M.L. (1990) Pregnancies from biopsied human preimplantation embryos sexed by Y-specific DNA amplification. *Nature* **344**: 768–770

Harper, J.C. & Handyside, A.H. (1994) The current status of preimplantation diagnosis. *Current Obstetrics and Gynaecology* **4**: 143–149.

Harper, J.C., Coonan, E. & Ramaekers, F.C.S. (1994) Identification of the sex of human preimplantation embryos in two hours using an improved spreading method and fluorescent in-situ hybridization (FISH) using directly labelled probes. *Human Reproduction* **9**: 721–724.

Harrison K., Wilson L., Breen T., Pope A., Cummins J. & Hennessy J. (1988) Fertilization of human oocytes in relation to varying delay before insemination. *Fertility and Sterility* **50**: 294–297.

Holst, N. (1990) Optimization and simplification of culture conditions in human in Vitro Fertilization (IVF) and pre-embryo replacement by serum-free media. *Journal of In Vitro Fertilization and Embryo Transfer*, **7**: 47–53.

Homberg, R. & Shelef, M. (1995) Factors affecting oocyte quality. In: *Gametes: the Oocyte* (Grudzinskao, J.G. & Yorich, J.L., eds), Cambridge University Press, pp. 227–291.

Howles, C.M., Macnamee, M.C. & Edwards, R.G. (1987) Follicular development and early luteal function of conception and non-conceptual cycles after human in vitro fertilization. *Human Reproduction* **2**: 17–21.

Khan, I., Staessen, C., Van den Abbeel, E., Camus, M., Wisanto, A., Smitz, J., Devroey, P. & Van Steirteghem, A.C. (1989) Time of insemination and its effect on in vitro fertilization, cleavage and pregnancy rates in GnRH agonist/HMG-stimulated cycles. *Human Reproduction* **4**: 531–535.

Kruger, T.F., Stander, F.S.H., Smith, K., Van Der Merue, J.P. & Lombard, C.J. (1987) The effect of serum supplementation on the cleavage of human embryos. *Journal of In Vitro Fertilization Embryo Transfer* **4**: 10.

Leese, H.J. (1987) Analysis of embryos by noninvasive methods. *Human Reproduction* **2**: 37–40.

Leung, P., Gronow, M., Kellow, G., Lopata, A., Spiers, A., McBain, J., du Plessis, Y. & Johnston, I. (1984) Serum supplement in human in vitro fertilisation and embryo development. *Fertility and Sterility* **41**: 36–917.

Levron, J., Munné, S., Willadsen, S., Rosenwaks, Z. & Cohen, J. (1995) Male and female genomes associated in a single pronucleus in human zygotes. *Journal of Assisted Reproduction and Genetics* **12** (Suppl.): 27s.

Lopata, A., Johnston, I.W.H., Hoult, I.J. & Speins, A.L. (1980) Pregnancy following intrauterine implantation of an embryo obtained by in vitro fertilization of a preovulatory egg. *Fertility and Sterility* **33**: 117.

Macnamee, M.C., Howles, C.M. & Edwards, R.G. (1989) Short term luteinising hormone agonist treatment: prospective trial of a novel ovarian stimulation regimen for in vitro fertilisation. *Fertility and Sterility* **52**: 264–269.

Marrs, R.P., Saito, H., Yee, B., Sato, F. & Brown, J. (1984) Effect of variation of in vitro culture techniques upon oocyte fertilization and embryo development in human in vitro fertilization procedures. *Fertility and Sterility* **41**: 519–523.

Menezo, Y., Guerin, J.F. & Czyba, J.C. (1990) Improvement of human early embryo development in vitro by coculture on monolayers of Vero cells. *Biological Reproduction* **42**: 301–305.

Menezo, Y., Dumont, M., Hazout, A., Nicollet, B., Pouly, J.L. & Janny, L. (1995) Culture and co-culture techniques. In: *Fertility and Sterility* (Hedon, Bringer, Mares, eds), IFFS-95, The Parthenon Publishing Group, pp. 413–418.

Menezo, Y., Hazout, A., Dumont, M., Herbaut, N. & Nicollet, B. (1992) Coculture of embryos on Vero cells and transfer of blastocyst in human. *Human Reproduction* **7**: 101–106.

Menezo, Y., Testart, J. & Perrone, D. (1984) Serum is not necessary in human in vitro fertilization, early embryo culture, and transfer. *Fertility and Sterility* **42**: 750.

Muggleton-Harris, A.L., Findlay, I. & Whittingham, D.G. (1990) Improvement of the culture conditions for the development of human preimplantation embryos. *Human Reproduction* **5**: 217–220.

Munné, S., Alikani, M., Levron, J., Tomkin, G., Palermo, G., Grifo, J. & Cohen, J. (1995) Fluorescent in situ hibridization in human blastomeres. In: *Fertility and Sterility* (Hedon, Bringer, Mares, eds), IFFS-95, The Parthenon Publishing Group, pp. 425–438.

Oehninger, S., Acosta, A.A., Veeck, L.L., Simonetti, S. & Muasher, S.J. (1989) Delayed fertilization during in vitro fertilization and embryo transfer cycles: analysis of cause and impact of overall results. *Fertility and Sterility* **52**: 991–997.

Pampiglione, J.S., Mills, C., Campbell, S., Steer, C., Kingsland, C. & Mason, B.A. (1990) The clinical outcome of reinsemination of human oocytes fertilized in vitro. *Fertility and Sterility* **53**: 306–310.

Pickering, S.J., Braude, P.R., Johnson, M.H., Cant, A. & Currie, J. (1990). Transient cooling to room temperature can cause irreversible disruption of the meiotic spindle in the human oocyte. *Fertility and Sterility* **54**: 102–108.

Plachot, M. & Mandelbaum, J. (1990) Oocyte maturation, fertilization and embryonic growth in vitro. *British Medical Bulletin* **46**: 675–694.

Plachot, M., Veiga, A. & Montagut, J. et al (1988) Are clinical and biological IVF parameters correlated with chromosomal disorders in early life: a multicentric study. *Human Reproduction* **3**: 627–635.

Plachot, M., de Grouchy, J., Montagut, J., Lepetre, S., Carle, E., Veiga, A., Calderon, G. & Santalo, J. (1987). Multi-centric study of chromosome analysis in human oocytes and embryos in an IVF programme. *Human Reproduction* **2**: 29.

Plachot, M., Mandelbaum, J., Junca, A.M., Cohen, J. & Salat-Baroux, J. (1993) Coculture of human embryos with granulosa cells. *Contracept. Fertil. Sex* **19**: 632–634.

Purdy, J.M. (1982) Methods for fertilization and embryo culture in vitro, In: *Human Conception In Vitro* (Edwards, R.G., Purdy, J.M. eds), Academic Press, London, p. 135.

Quinn, P., Warner, G.M., Klein, J.E. & Kirby, C. (1985) Culture factors affecting the success rate of in vitro fertilization and embryo transfer. *Annals of the New York Academy of Sciences* **412**: 195.

Regan, L., Owen, E.J. & Jacobs, H.S. (1990) Hypersecretion of luteinising hormone, infertility, and miscarriage. *Lancet* **336**: 1141–1144.

Rinehart, J.S., Bavister, B.D. & Gerrity, M. (1988) Quality control in the in vitro fertilization laboratory: comparison of bioassay systems for water quality. *Journal of In Vitro Fertilization and Embryo Transfer* **5**: 335–425.

Roert, J., Verhoeff, A., van Lent, M., Hisman, G.J. & Zeilmaker, G.H. (1995) Results of decentralised in vitro fertilization treatment with transport and satellite clinics. *Human Reproduction* **10**: 563–567.

Saito, H., Berger T., Mishell, D.R. Jr & Marrs, R.P. (1984) The effect of serum fractions on embryo growth. *Fertility and Sterility* **41**: 761–765.

Shaw, J., Harrison, K., Wilson, L., Breen, T., Shaw, G., Cummins, J. & Hennessey, J. (1987) Results using medium supplemented with either fresh or frozen serum in human in vitro fertilization. *Journal of In Vitro Fertilization Embryo Transfer* **3:** 215–217.

Staessen, C., Van den Abbeel, E., Carle, Ml, Khan, I., Devroey, P. & Van Steirteghem, A.C. (1990) Comparison between human serum and Albuminar-20 (TM) supplement for in vitro fertilization. *Human Reproduction* **5:** 336–341.

Veeck, L.L. (1986) Insemination and fertilization. In: *In Vitro Fertilization – Norfolk* (Jones, H.W., Jr, Jones, G.S., Hodgen, G.D., Rosenwaks, Z. eds), Williams & Wilkins, Baltimore, p. 183.

Veeck, L.L. (1988) Oocyte assessment and biological performance. *Annals of the New York Academy of Sciences of the USA* **541:** 259–262.

Weimer. K.E., Hoffman, D.I., Maxon, W.S., Eager, S., Muhlberger, R., Fior, I. & Cuervo, M. (1993) Embryonic morphology and rate of implantation of human embryos following co-culture on bovine oviductal epithelial cells. *Human Reproduction* **8:** 97–101.

11
Cryopreservation

Embryo freezing and thawing

Following fresh embryo transfer in a stimulated IVF cycle, supernumerary embryos suitable for cryopreservation are available in a large number of cycles. During the period 1990–96, 60% of stimulated in vitro fertilization (IVF) cycles at Bourn Hall Clinic had supernumerary embryos cryopreserved. Successful cryopreservation of zygotes and embryos has greatly enhanced the clinical benefits and cumulative conception rate possible for a couple following a single cycle of ovarian stimulation and IVF. Other clear benefits include the possibility of avoiding fresh embryo transfer in stimulated cycles with a potential for ovarian hyperstimulation syndrome, or in which factors which may jeopardize implantation are apparent, (e.g. bleeding, unfavourable endometrium, polyps, or extremely difficult embryo transfer).

The first live births following frozen-thawed embryo transfer were reported in 1984 and 1985 by groups in Australia, The Netherlands, and UK and since then the original protocols have been modified and simplified such that cryopreservation as an adjunct to a routine IVF programme may lead to successful

---

Contraindications to Fresh Embryo Transfer

- Risk of ovarian hyperstimulation syndrome (OHSS)
- Intermenstrual bleeding
- Poor quality endometrium
- Uterine polyp
- Poor uterine perfusion measured by doppler studies

   Proceed with OCR and insemination, cryopreserve all embryos for transfer in a subsequent cycle

survival of up to 80% of the embryos frozen, with subsequent pregnancy and live birth rates of 28% and 22%, respectively (at Bourn Hall Clinic). Although the routine protocols required are simple and easily undertaken, an understanding of the basic principles of cryobiology involved is essential to ensure that the methodology is correctly and successfully applied to minimize cell damage during the processes of freezing and thawing. There are physicochemical consequences as a result of direct temperature effects, and as a result of the effect of ice formation. The presence of appropriate concentrations of cryoprotectant solution, and controlled rates of cooling and warming are important factors in determining optimum survival.

Exposing a cell to a reduction in its physiological temperature has effects at several different levels.

1. The biochemistry of metabolic processes is altered and disrupted: some enzymes are destabilized, and there may be a loss of ions from cell organelles as well as from the cell itself. Active transport mechanisms are affected.
2. Lipid–protein complexes are very vulnerable during cooling. Unlike simple proteins which are held together by strong covalent bonds, they are held by much weaker associations. The high sensitivity of these lipid–protein complexes to profound changes in the physicochemical environment may result in irreversible damage to the cell membranes unless care is taken to preserve their integrity.
3. A fall in temperature results in increased gas solubility, allowing the formation of intracytoplasmic gas bubbles which disrupt intracellular organization and destroy organelles upon thawing.
4. With decreasing temperature and ice formation, less water is available as a solvent for the remaining salts, with a resulting increase in osmotic pressure producing dehydration and membrane stress. The buffering capacity of the medium alters as bicarbonate and sodium chloride precipitate out of solution.
5. When the eutectic point of the solution is reached, consequent ice formation, 'supercooling', results in the liberation of heat of fusion which interrupts the programmed linear fall in temperature. This fluctuation has a dramatic effect upon cell survival, and must be overcome with controlled induction of ice crystal formation at a temperature of -6 to $-7\,°C$ by 'seeding'. This precipitates a nucleus of ice, overcoming the effects due to the liberation of latent heat of fusion.

Low molecular weight cryoprotective solutes help to protect the cells by reducing the quantity of ice formed intracellularly. Sucrose acts as both a dehydrating agent and an osmotic buffer, minimizing the potential for intracellular ice formation and osmotic damage. A controlled slow rate of cooling with the use of a programmed cell freezer permits remaining cytoplasmic water to flow out of the cell and freeze extracellularly, with gradual cell dehydration. If cool-

134 *Cryopreservation*

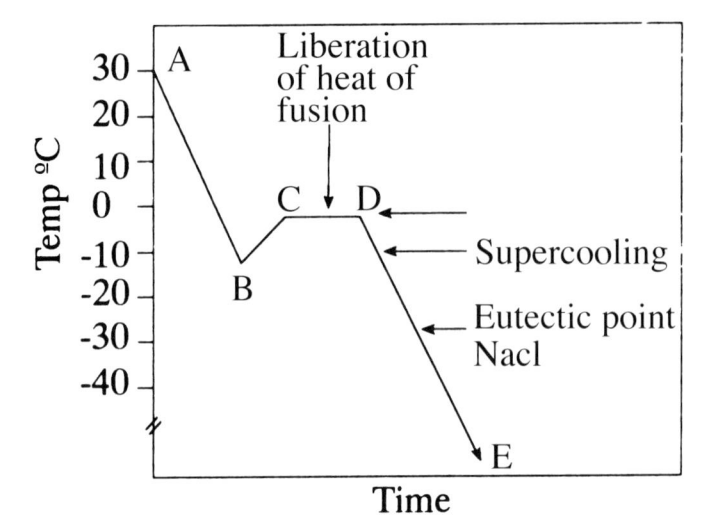

Figure 11.1 Graph showing temperature changes during programmed cell freezing, with release of latent heat of fusion at the eutectic point.

Embryo Cryopreservation

Select only good quality embryos for freezing
- Pronucleate: intact zona pellucida

  clean healthy cytoplasm

  two distinct pronuclei visible

Do not freeze zygotes which are progressing into syngamy
- Cleavage: regular blastomeres with less than 20% fragments

---

ing is too rapid, the cytoplasm will not have enough time to dehydrate and will eventually freeze with the formation of intracellular ice leading to cell damage and death upon thawing. The optimal rate of cooling differs for different cell types, and is related to cell volume and surface area, water permeability, Arrhenius activation energy, and the type and concentration of cryoprotectant additives used (Figure 11.1).

Three different cryoprotectants have been successfully used for human embryo cryopreservation: dimethyl sulphoxide (DMSO), glycerol, and 1,2-propanediol. Propanediol is less toxic than DMSO, with better cell penetration; the protocol presented by Lasalle and Testart in 1985 described here has consistently yielded 70–80% survival rates and 12% implantation rate per embryo transferred in routine use at Bourn Hall Clinic over the past ten years.

Embryo selection for cryopreservation

Using 1,2-propanediol as cryoprotectant, embryos can be frozen at either the pronucleate or early cleavage stages. Careful selection of viable embryos with a good prognosis for survival is paramount in achieving acceptable success rates.

1. *Pronucleate:* The cell must have an intact zona pellucida, and healthy cytoplasm with two distinct pronuclei clearly visible. Accurate timing of zygote freezing is essential to avoid periods of the cell cycle which are highly sensitive to cooling. During the period when pronuclei start to migrate before syngamy with DNA synthesis and formation of the mitotic spindle, the microtubular system is highly vulnerable to temperature fluctuation, leading to scattering of the chromosomes. Zygotes processed for freezing at this stage will no longer survive cryopreservation. The timing of pronucleate freezing is crucial, and the process must be initiated while the pronuclei are still distinctly apparent: normally from 20 to 22 hours after insemination.
2. *Cleavage:* 2–8 cell embryos must be of good quality, Grade 1 or 2, with less than 20% cytoplasmic fragments. Uneven blastomeres and a high degree of fragmentation jeopardize survival potential.

Media preparation

MATERIALS

Phosphate buffered saline (PBS) – Gibco Ltd, PO Box 35, Paisley, Scotland.
1,2-Propanediol (PROH) – Sigma (Propylene glycol)
Sucrose

Freezing solutions

1. 100 ml (PBS, Gibco)
2. 1.5 M PROH
   86.3 ml PBS
   13.7 ml PROH (agitate gently as you add)
3. 1.5 M PROH/0.1 M sucrose
   86.3 ml PBS
   13.7 ml PROH (agitate gently)
   4.1 g sucrose (allow to dissolve)

Thawing solutions

1. 1.0 M PROH + 0.2 M Sucrose
   90.9 ml PBS

>   9.1 ml PROH (agitate gently)
>   8.2 g sucrose (allow to dissolve)
> 2. 0.5 M PROH + 0.2 M sucrose
>   Use a 1:1 mixture of (1) & (3)
> 3. 0.2 M Sucrose
>   100 ml PBS
>   8.2 g sucrose
> 4. PBS

Optional: Phenol red may be added to each solution as a colourant: add 0.2 ml Phenol red to each 100 ml of solution.

After preparation the solutions are filtered through a 0.22 μm Millipore filter, labelled, and stored in 10 ml sterile aliquots at room temperature in the dark.

Working solutions: + 20% serum. Add 0.2 ml human serum albumin to each 1 ml of solution immediately before use.

Method

Details of each patient and embryos must be carefully recorded on appropriate data sheets. Meticulous and complete record keeping is crucial, and must include the patient's date of birth, medical number, date of oocyte retrieval (OCR), date of cryopreservation, number and type of embryos frozen, together with clear and accurate identification of storage vessel and location within the storage vessel.

Handle the preselected embryos with fire-polished clean sterile pasteur pipettes, using a different pipette for each patient. Fine glass probes may also be required, to help in locating the embryos within their dishes or wells.

> 1. Use 1 ml aliquots of each solution per patient, and add 20% human serum albumin just before use to make the working solutions.
> 2. Warm the solutions to 37 °C
> 3. Prepare labelled dishes, either 3 × 35 mm petri dishes per patient, or one 4-well Nunc plate per patient.
> 4. Transfer embryos and warmed solutions to room temperature: the embryos are transferred initially to the first solution at 37 °C, and thereafter allowed to cool gradually to room temperature. Pipette the embryos:

> 1. F1 (PBS + 20% serum): wash to remove traces of medium, then pipette into
> 2. F2 (PBS + serum + 1.5m M PROH): leave to equilibrate at room temperature, 15 minutes
> 3. F3 (PBS + serum + PROH + 0.1 M sucrose): leave for 10–15 minutes at room temperature

Embryo freezing and thawing 137

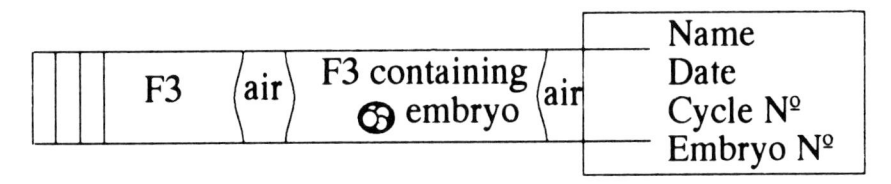

Figure 11.2 Loading embryos into a cryostraw before freezing.

4. Load into pre-labelled straws or ampoules. Straws: IMV BP 81 L'Aigle, France. Paillette Cristal 91, Ref. ZA 180. Distributed by Rocket-Medical, Imperial Way, Watford WD2 4XX, UK.

Loading into straws:
Attach a 1 ml syringe with appropriate silicon tubing adaptor to the straw, and fill as follows:
2 cm F3 solution, followed by 1 cm air, then 2 cm F3 containing the embryo (one per straw) followed by air to draw the first volume of F3 into the polyvinyl chloride (PVC) plug, creating a seal. The other end of the straw can be sealed with a pre-labelled colour-coded plug. Each straw must be clearly identifiable with precise patient details including name, date of birth, record number, and date of freezing (Figure 11.2).

Ampoules:
Tissue-culture washed Borosilicate glass ampoules with a fine-drawn neck can be used. First fill the ampoule with approximately 0.4 ml of the sucrose/PROH solution using a needle and syringe, then carefully transfer the embryos using a fine-drawn Pasteur pipette. Using a high-intensity flame, carefully heat-seal the neck of the ampoule. It is important to ensure (under the microscope) that the seal is complete, without leaks: leakage of liquid nitrogen into the ampoule during freezing will cause it to explode immediately upon thawing!

Freezing programme: (Planer Kryo 10)

Switch on the programmed cell freezer and ensure that the liquid nitrogen level is sufficient for 2–3 hours of use.
Start temperature: 20 °C

      Ramp 1: -1 °C/min to 19.8 °C
      Ramp 2: Hold 00.05 (5 minutes, to complete loading of straws or ampoules into the machine)
      Ramp 3: -2° C/min to −7 °C
      Soak time: 00.05 (5 minutes)

Manual seeding is carried out at −6.5 °C
   Ramp 4: −0.3 °C/min to −31 °C
   Ramp 5: −50 °C/min to −160 °C

Hold: 01.00 (10 minutes) to allow unloading and plunging into liquid nitrogen.

Embryo Cryopreservation - Method

- Wash in phosphate buffered saline + 20% serum
- Transfer to 1 ml of 1.5 M Propanediol (PROH) + 20% serum
  leave for 15 minutes at room temperature
- Transfer to 1 ml of 1.5 M PROH + 0.1M sucrose + 20% serum
  leave for 10–15 minutes at room temperature
- Load into ampoules or straws, transfer to programmed cell freezer

---

IMPORTANT: Seeding should be performed at −6.5 °C. Use a liquid nitrogen cooled spatula, forceps or cotton bud to touch the surface of each straw, or cooled forceps encircling the meniscus of the glass ampoule. Remove the implement as soon as ice formation is seen, otherwise the temperature change in the immediate vicinity of the nucleation will be lower than anticipated. Before the programme finishes, everything should be ready so that the embryos can be plunged directly into liquid nitrogen. Hold pre-labelled colour-coded plastic goblets (Visitubes, Rocket Medical) under liquid nitrogen using clamp forceps, transfer the straws or ampoules immediately into the appropriate liquid nitrogen-containing goblet, and then transfer the goblet to the pre-allocated and recorded space in a storage Dewar.

Thawing

Prepare:

1. 30 °C water bath for straws, or 37 °C water bath for ampoules
2. Labelled petri dishes or Nunc plate
3. Thawing solutions at room temperature
4. Fire-polished sterile Pasteur pipettes and probe
5. Patient freeze/thaw data sheet.

The thawing protocol is carried out at room temperature, and the embryos placed in equilibrated culture medium at room temperature before being allowed to warm gradually to 37°C in the incubator.

1. Remove straws or ampoules from liquid nitrogen
2. i) Straws: Hold at room temperature 40 seconds
   Wipe with a dry tissue to remove excess ice
   Plunge into 30 °C waterbath for 1 minute.
   Remove the plug from the straw(s) and release the embryos into the first thawing solution (1.0 M PROH, 0.2 M sucrose).
   ii) Ampoules: thaw in 37 °C waterbath.
   Using a fine-drawn pipette, aspirate and decant the contents of the ampoule into the petri dish or well.
   Identify the embryo(s) under the microscope, and transfer to solution Tl.
3. Leave for 5 minutes.
4. Transfer to T2 (PBS + 20% serum + 0.5 M PROH + 0.2 M sucrose), 5 minutes.
5. Transfer to T3 (PBS + 20% serum + 0.2 M sucrose), 5 minutes.
6. Wash in PBS (T4) and then transfer through two wash drops or wells of culture medium before placing the embryos in their final culture drop or well.
7. Incubate at 37 °C. in the CO_2 incubator until the time of embryo transfer.

Pronucleate embryos are cultured overnight to ensure that the zygotes continue development, and transferred only if cleavage takes place.

Cleavage stage embryos are incubated for a minimum of 1 hour before transfer.

Embryo Thawing

Rapid thaw to 30° C
Incubate at room temperature in
- 1.0 M PROH/0.2 M Sucrose + 20% serum   5 minutes
- 0.5 M PROH/0.2 M Sucrose + 20% serum   5 minutes
- 0.2 M Sucrose + 20% serum   5 minutes

Wash through 3 drops of culture medium
Incubate at 37° C:
      Pronucleate: incubate overnight to assess cleavage
      Cleaved: incubate at least 1 hour

Blastocyst freezing

Although the same propanediol protocol has recently been applied to the freezing of blastocysts, they can also be successfully frozen using glycerol in a final concentration of 9%. Prepare culture dishes containing two drops of each glycerol dilution under a layer of equilibrated oil (or four-well plates containing two aliquots of each glycerol dilution), and equilibrate the dishes to 37 °C in the

CO_2 incubator. The addition and removal of glycerol should be carried out at or near 37 °C rather than at room temperature.

Make dilutions to final concentrations of:

a) Freezing: 1. 5% glycerol (v/v) in culture medium, 10 minutes.
2. 9% glycerol (v/v) in culture medium containing 0.2 M Sucrose, 10 minutes.

b) Thawing: 1. 0.5 M Sucrose in culture medium, 10 minutes.
2. 0.2 M Sucrose in culture medium, 10 minutes.
3. Wash through 2–3 drops or aliquots of culture medium and replace in culture.

Planer Kryo 10 programme for blastocyst freezing

Start temperature 20 °C.
1. −1 °C/min to 19.8 °C.
2. Hold 00.05 (minutes)
3. −1 °C/min to −7 °C
Soak time 00.05 for seeding
4. −0.30 °C/min to −37.0°C
5. Hold 01.00 – plunge into liquid nitrogen

Manual seeding at −6.5 °C.
Soak time 00.05

Planer Kryo 10 operation

1. Ensure that there is an adequate level of liquid nitrogen in the Dewar, leaving an air space. The container should not be more than two-thirds full. Immerse the probe and attach the pressure gauge securely. Close the red toggle switch on the pressure gauge.
2. Switch power on, and pressurize the system by pressing the white switch on the platform. An orange indicator light should appear and extinguishes automatically when the correct pressure is reached (5–7.5 psi).
3. Press RUN/HOLD. The display will prompt 'Enter access level 1'
4. Enter password: 3333
5. Display prompts: 'Which programme?' Use arrow keys to alter, select programme and press ENTER.
6. Display reads 'Programme Start 20 °C'
7. Press RUN. Ramp 1 will lead to starting temperature, and alarm will sound when it is reached. Display reads 'Load Samples'.
8. Load samples and press RUN.

9. When seeding temperature is reached, the alarm sounds and the machine will hold the temperature at −6.5 °C. SEED all the samples, then press RUN. The machine continues the programme to Ramp 5.
10. Before the end of the programme, prepare a small vessel of liquid nitrogen containing prelabelled plastic goblets, held under the nitrogen with artery forceps. At the end of the programme, remove all the samples and plunge them directly into the liquid nitrogen filled goblets.
11. Transfer the samples to their pre-selected storage space, and confirm the recorded position on appropriate embryo storage records.

IMPORTANT: Seeding must be performed whilst the chamber is at -6.5 to -7°C. Use a liquid nitrogen cooled spatula or forceps to touch the meniscus at the top of the column of liquid, and replace the sample in the chamber immediately.

12. To switch off, or abort a run:
    Press 5: display prompts 'ENTER to confirm', press ENTER.
    Display reads 'Run, chamber temp = ... °C'
    Press RUN
    Display reads 'Do not switch off'
    When ambient temperature is reached, display reads 'ready to restart'
    Switch power off
    Open the toggle switch on the Dewar to release the pressure

During a run, the display can be altered using arrow keys to show: time left for that segment, demand temperature, ramp end temperature, ramp rate, name and no. of programme, chamber temperature.

Clinical aspects of frozen embryo transfer

Freeze-thawed embryos must be transferred to a uterus which is optimally receptive for implantation, post-ovulation. Patients with regular ovulatory cycles and an adequate luteal phase may have their embryos transferred in a natural cycle, monitored by ultrasound and blood or urine luteinizing hormone (LH) levels in order to pinpoint ovulation. Embryo transfer is routinely carried out three days after the onset of the LH surge, i.e. 2 days post-ovulation.

Older patients, or those with irregular cycles may have their embryos transferred in an artificial cycle with the administration of hormone replacement therapy using exogenous steroids after creating an artificial menopause by downregulation with a luteinizing hormone releasing hormone (LHRH) agonist.

Transfer in a natural menstrual cycle

1. Patient selection
    regular cycles, 28 ± 3 days
    previously assay luteal phase progesterone to confirm ovulation
2. Cycle monitoring
    from day 10 until ovulation is confirmed, by:
        daily ultrasound scan
        daily plasma LH (± oestradiol, progesterone)
3. Be prepared to cancel if
    peak oestradiol is < 650 pmol/L
    endometrial thickness is < 8 mm at the time of LH surge
4. Timing of embryo transfer
    pronucleate embryos:
        thaw on day 1 after ovulation (LH + 3)
        culture overnight before transfer.

    cleavage stage embryos:
        thaw and transfer on day 2 after ovulation
        (LH + 4)

    blastocysts:
        thaw and transfer on day 4 after ovulation
        (LH + 6)

Patients with irregular cycles may be induced to ovulate using clomiphene citrate or gonadotrophins, and embryo transfer timed in relation either to the endogenous LH surge or following administration of human chorionic gonadotrophin (hCG).

Transfer in an artificial cycle

1. Patient selection: oligomenorrhoea/irregular cycles,
    age > 38 years
2. Downregulate with LHRH analogue (buserelin or nafarelin) for at least 14 days, continue downregulation until the time of embryo transfer
3. Oestradiol valerate days 1–5   2 mg
                              6–9   4 mg
                              10–13   6 mg
                              14 onwards 4 mg
4. Progesterone:
    day 15–16   Gestone 50 mg intramuscular (Ferring)

or cyclogest pessaries 200 mg twice daily (Cyclogest, Hoechst)

or utrogestan pessaries 100 mg three times daily (Utrogestan, Besins-Iscovesco)

and double dose from day 17 onwards

(100 mg Gestone, 400 mg twice daily cyclogest, 200 mg three times daily utrogestan)

5. Embryo transfer:

Pronucleate: thaw on day 16 of the artificial cycle, culture overnight before transfer on day 17.

Cleavage stage embryos: thaw and replace on day 17.

6. If pregnancy is established, continue hormone replacement (HRT) therapy:

8 mg oestradiol valerate

higher dose of progesterone supplement daily until day 77 after embryo transfer; then gradually withdraw the drugs with monitoring of blood P4 (progesterone) levels.

This protocol is also successfully used for the treatment of agonadal women who require ovum or embryo donation. In combination with prior gonadotrophin releasing hormone (GnRH) pituitary suppression, the artificial cycle can be timed to a pre-scheduled programme according to the patient's (or clinic's) convenience.

Results

In a series of 1009 FER cycles at Bourn Hall Clinic from 1991 to 1994, the clinical pregnancy rates using the different transfer regimens can be seen in Table 11.1:

Table 11.1

	Number	No. pregnant (%)
All cycles	1009	259 (26)
Natural cycles	421	35 (32)
HRT cycles	588	124 (21)
Freeze all embryos	290	110 (38)
Surplus embryos only	719	149 (21)
Cleaving embryos	241	44 (18)
Pronucleate embryos	768	215 (28)

Notes:
HRT: hormone replacement therapy.
Clinical pregnancy rates (viable gestation sacs per embryo transfer procedure) after frozen-thawed embryo transfer at Bourn Hall Clinic from 1991 to 1994

Oocyte cryopreservation

Many of the legal and ethical problems created by the cryopreservation and storage of embryos might be overcome by preserving oocytes. In addition, for young women about to undergo treatment for malignant disease which will result in loss of ovarian function, oocyte cryopreservation would provide them with a means of preserving their own genetic material prior to treatment, giving them the hope of having their own family in the future. Although a few pregnancies after oocyte freeze-thawing and fertilization were reported in the mid-1980s, oocyte survival and fertilization rates have been poor, and to the present date oocyte cryopreservation has not been introduced into routine clinical practice.

In the mouse system, high rates of aneuploidy following oocyte freeze-thawing were observed, thought to arise from abnormalities of the spindle apparatus which is highly temperature sensitive and depolymerizes with temperature reduction. Promising reports of successful human oocyte cryopreservation are this year (1996) starting to appear in the literature, using the identical propanediol/sucrose slow freeze/rapid thaw method described above for embryo cryopreservation. Optimum success rates were obtained in combination with intracytoplasmic sperm injection (ICSI) instead of normal insemination of oocytes, and a few clinics are now beginning to offer oocyte cryopreservation on a clinical basis, although the number of pregnancies reported still remains in single figures so far.

Semen cryopreservation

Semen can be successfully cryopreserved using either glycerol alone, or a complex cryoprotective medium as cryoprotectant. Cooling and freezing can be carried out by using a programmed cell freezer, or by simply suspending the prepared specimens in liquid nitrogen vapour for a period of 30 minutes.

Cryopreserved semen has long been used successfully for artificial insemination, intrauterine insemination, and IVF. When it is to be used for intrauterine insemination or IVF, the sample must be carefully washed or prepared by density gradient centrifugation to remove all traces of cryoprotectant medium. Although freeze-thawing does produce damage to the cells with loss of up to 50% of pre-freeze motility, the large numbers of cells available can still achieve successful fertilization even with low cryosurvival rates. There is, however, a noticeable difference in cryosurvival rates between normal semen and semen with abnormal parameters such as low count and motility, and samples from men who require sperm cryopreservation prior to chemotherapy treatment for malignant disease frequently show very poor cryosurvival rates. The now routine introduction of ICSI into IVF practice has overcome this problem, so that successful fertilization using ICSI is possible even with extremely poor cryosurvival of suboptimal samples.

Sample preparation

Samples should be prepared and frozen within 1-2 hours of ejaculation.

1. Perform semen analysis according to standard laboratory technique, and label two plastic conical tubes and an appropriate number of 0.5 ml freezing straws or ampoules for each specimen. Record all details on appropriate record sheets.
2. Add small aliquots of cryoprotectant medium (CPM) to the semen at room temperature over a period of 2 minutes, to a ratio of 1:1.
   If the ejaculate volume is greater than 5 ml, divide the sample into two aliquots before mixing with CPM.
3. Aliquot the diluted sample into straws or ampoules, labelling aliquots for assessment of post-thaw count and motility.
4. Dilute specimens with CPM according to count.
   60 million/ml   dilute 1:1 semen:/CPM
   20 – 60 million/ml   dilute 2:1 semen:/CPM
   20 million/ml   dilute 4:1 semen:/CPM
5. Re-assess the number of motile sperm/ml, which should ideally be 10 million or above.
6. Aliquot into pre-labelled straws.

Manual freezing

1. Place the ampoules or straws (in goblets) on a metal cane
2. Refrigerate at 4 °C for 15 minutes
3. Place into liquid nitrogen vapour for 25 minutes
4. Plunge into liquid nitrogen for storage, and record storage details.

Kryo-10 semen freezing programme

1. Start temperature 24 °C (room temperature)
2. Cooling: -2 °C per minute to 0 °C.
3. $\qquad$ -10.0 °C. per minute to -100 °C.
4. HOLD: 10 minutes (total programme time = 37 minutes)
5. Transfer to liquid nitrogen flask for temporary storage before placing in liquid phase of cryostorage tank.
6. Record all storage details appropriately.

7. Assess post-thaw motility: thaw straws at 34 °C. Wipe the outside to remove debris and condensation, snip both ends with scissors, dicard one or two drops of the sample, and assess the sample for count and motility.

% Cryosurvival = (post-thaw motility/pre-freeze motility)×100

Insemination

Intracervical: after thawing, aspirate the semen with a 2 ml syringe and a Kwill five inch filling tube. Insemination should be carried out immediately, as frozen-thawed sperm do not remain active for as long as fresh sperm.

Intrauterine: process the thawed sample on a discontinuous density gradient, wash, and resuspend in 0.5–1 ml of culture medium before loading into the appropriate catheter for insemination.

Cryoprotective medium (CPM)

Primary Stock Solutions:

1. Sodium Citrate ($Na_3(C_6H_5O)\,2H_2O$) 0.1 N
   Primary buffer (PB)
   dissolve 8.82 g sodium citrate in 300 ml distilled water.
2. Glucose ($C_6H_2O_6$) 0.33 M
   Primary glucose (PG)
   dissolve 5.46 g glucose in 100 ml distilled water.
3. Fructose($C_6H_{12}O_6$) 0.33 M
   Primary fructose (PF)
   dissolve 5.4 g fructose in 100 ml distilled water.

Filter through a 0.22 μm Millipore filter and store in sterile containers at 4 °C.

Secondary buffer (KSB)

KSB buffer is used in the final preparation of CPM and has a 1 month storage life at +5 °C.

It is composed of 3 parts PB:1 part PG:1 part PF,
  i.e. 300 ml PB:100 ml PG:100 ml PF.
Mix thoroughly.

Storage

Aliquots of KSB can be frozen with glycerol added:
  13 ml KSB + 3 ml glycerol.
Store in sterile containers (e.g. 50 ml Falcon flasks) at −20 °C.

Final CPM preparation

KSB	13 ml	65% by volume
Glycerol	3 ml	15% by volume
Egg yolk	4 ml	20% by volume

1. Thaw frozen KSB/glycerol mixture
2. Obtain the yolk from a fresh free range egg and separate it from the white by carefully rolling the isolated yolk on filter paper.
   Using a sterile disposable syringe and needle, withdraw the required volume from the yolk sac.
   It is important to ensure that the aliquot of egg yolk is free of egg white albumin.
3. Add egg yolk to KSB and glycerol and mix thoroughly.
4. Heat inactivate at 56 °C for 30 minutes and then cool.
5. Add glycine : 200 mg/20 ml CPM
6. Adjust pH of CPM to pH 7.2–.3 using 0.1 N NaOH or 1.3% $NaHCO_3$ solution.
7. CPM can be stored at 4 °C for 10 days.

Further reading

Al-Hasani, S., Ludwig, M., Diedrich,. K., Bauer, O., Kipker, W., Diedrich, Ch., Sturm, R. & Yilmaz, A.(1996) Preliminary results on the incidence of polyploidy in cryopreserved human oocytes after ICSI. *Human Reproduction* **11**: Abstract book 1, 50–51.

Ashwood-Smith, M.J. (1986) The cryopreservation of human embryos. *Human Reproduction* **1**; 319–332.

Avery, S.M., Spillane, S., Marcus, S., Macnamee, M. & Brinsden, P. (1995) Factors affecting the outcome of frozen embryo replacement – experience of 1009 cycles. Presented at 15th World Congress on Fertility and Sterility, Montpelier. Abstract no. S6/0C.023.

Cohen J., Devane, G.W., Elsner C.W., Fehilly, C.B., Kort, H.I., Massey, J.B. & Turner, T.G. (1988) Cryopreservation of zygotes and early cleaved human embryos. *Fertility and Sterility* **49**: 2.

Cohen, J., Simons, R.F., Edwards, R.G., Fehilly, C.B. & Fishel, S.B. (1985) Pregnancies following the frozen storage of expanding human blastocysts. *Journal of In Vitro Fertilization and Embryo transfer* **2**: 59–64.

Fehilly, C.B., Cohen, J., Simons, R.F., Fishel, S.B. & Edwards, R.G. (1985) Cryopreservation of cleaving embryos and expanded blastocysts in the human: a comparative study. *Fertility and Sterility* **44**: 638–644.

Gook, D.A. (1996) Oocyte time-travel . . . can eggs arrive safely? *Alpha newsletter*, vol. 6, June 1996.

Gook, D.A., Osborn, S.M., Bourne, H. & Johnston, W.I.H. (1994) Fertilization of human oocytes following cryopreservation: normal karyotypes and absence of stray chromosomes. *Human Reproduction* **9**: 684–691.

Gook, D.A., Osborn, S.M. & Johnston, W.I.H. (1993) Cryopreservation of mouse and human oocytes using 1,2–propanediol and the configuration of the meiotic spindle. *Human Reproduction* **8**: 1101–1109.

Gook, D.A., Osborn, S.M. & Johnston, W.I.H (1995) Parthenogenetic activation of human oocytes following cryopreservation using 1,2–propanediol. *Human Reproduction* **10**: 654–658.

Gook, D.A., Schiewe, M.C., Osborn, S.M., Asch, R.H., Jansen, R.P.S. & Johnston, W.I.H. (1995) Intracytoplasmic sperm injection and embryo deveopment of human oocytes cryopreserved using 1,2–propanediol. *Human Reproduction* **10**: 2637–2641.

Hammerstedt, R.H., Graham, J.K. & Nolan, J.P. (1990) Cryopreservation of human sperm. *Journal of Andrology* 11, **1**: 73–88.

Hartshorne, G.M., Elder, K., Crow, J., Dyson, H. & Edwards, R.G. (1991). The influence of in vitro development upon post-thaw survival and implantation of cryopreserved human blastocycts. *Human Reproduction* **6**: 136–141.

Hartshorne, G.M., Wick, K., Elder, K. & Dyson, H. (1990) Effect of cell number at freezing upon survival and viability of cleaving embryos generated from stimulated IVF cycles. *Human Reproduction* **5**: 857–861.

Lassalle, B,, Testart, J., Renard, J.P. (1985) Human embryo features that influence the success of cryopreservation with the use of 1, 2, propanediol. *Fertility and Sterility* **44**: 645–651.

Lutjen, P., Trouson, A., Leeton, J., Findlay, J., Wood, C. & Renou, P. (1984) The establishment and maintenance of pregnancy using in vitro fertilization and embryo donation in a patient with primary ovarian failure. *Nature* **307**: 174.

McLaughlin, E.A., Ford, W.C.L. & Hill, M.G.R. (1990) A comparison of the freezing of human semen in the uncirculated vapour above liquid nitrogen and in a commercial semi-programmable freezer. *Human Reproduction* **5**: 734–738.

Mahadevan, M. & Trounson, A. (1983) Effects of CPM and dilution methods on the preservation of human spermatozoa. *Andrologia* **15**: 355–366.

Mazur, P. (1970) Cryobiology: the freezing of living systems. *Science* **168**: 93–949.

Mazur, P. (1984) Freezing of living cells: mechanisms and implications. *American Journal of Physiology* **247**: 125–142.

Pickering, S.J., Braude, P.R., Johnson, M.H., Cant, A. & Currie, J. (1990).Transient cooling to room temperature can cause irreversible disruption of the meiotic spindle in the human oocyte. *Fertility and Sterility* **54**: 102–108.12.

Ragni, G. & Vegetti, W. (1995) Cryopreservation of Semen. In: *Fertility and Sterility: a Current Overview.* (Hedon, Bringer, Mares, eds), The Parthenon Publishing Group, UK

Salat-Baroux, J., Cornet, D., Alvarez, S., Antoine, J.M., Tibi, C., Mandelbaum, J. & Plachot, M. (1988) Pregnancies after replacement of frozen-thawed embryos in a donation program. *Fertility and Sterility* **49**: 817–821.

Sathanandan, M., Macnamee, M.C., Wick, K. & Matthews, C.D. (1991) Clinical aspects of human embryo cryopreservation. In: *A Textbook of In Vitro Fertilization and Assisted Reproduction* (Brinsden, Rainsbury, eds), The Parthenon Publishing Group, UK

Schmidt, C.L., Taney, F.H., de Ziegler, D., Kuhar, M.J., Gagliardi, C.L., Colon, J.M., Mellon, R.W. & Weiss, G. (1989) Transfer of cryopreserved-thawed embryos: the natural cycle versus controlled preparation of the endometrium with gonadotropin-releasing hormone agonist and exogenous estnadiol and progesterone (GEEP). *Fertility and Sterility* **52**: 1609–1616.

Testart, J., Belaisch Allart, J., Lassalle, B., Hazout, A., Foreman, R., Rainhorn, J-D., Gazengel, A. & Frydman, R. (1987) Factors influencing the success rate of human embryo freezing in an in vitro fertilization and embryo transfer program. *Fertility and Sterility* **48**: 107–112.

Trounson, A. & Mohr, L. (1983). Human pregnancy following cryopreservation, thawing, and transfer of an eight-cell embryo. *Nature* **305:** 707–709.

Smith, A.U. (1952) Behaviour of fertilized rabbit eggs exposed to glycerol and to low temperatures. *Nature* **170:** 373.

Whittingham, D.G., Leibo, S.P. & Mazur, P. (1972) Survival of mouse embryos frozen to $-196\,°C$. and $-269\,°C$. *Science* **178:** 411–414.

12
Micromanipulation techniques

Intracytoplasmic sperm injection

Patient selection: indications for treatment

Until recently, the majority of cases of severe male factor infertility were virtually untreatable, and failure of fertilization was observed in up to 30% of in vitro fertilization–embryo transfer (IVF-ET) treatments for male infertility. The introduction of micromanipulation techniques such as zona drilling (ZD), partial zona dissection (PZD), and subzonal sperm injection (SUZI) raised the hopes of a better prognosis for these cases, but did not overall provide a substantial improvement in success rates. The introduction and successful application of intracytoplasmic sperm injection by the team led by Professor Van Steirteghem at The Free University in Brussels, Belgium, has produced a dramatic improvement in the treatment of severe male infertility by assisted reproductive technology.

The ICSI (intracytoplasmic sperm injection) procedure involves the injection of a single sperm cell directly into an oocyte, and it therefore can be used not only for cases in which there are extremely low numbers of sperm, but in bypassing gamete interaction at the level of the zona pellucida and the vitelline membrane, it can also be used in the treatment of qualitative or functional sperm disorders.

1. Couples who have suffered recurrent failure of fertilization after IVF-ET may have one or more disorders of gamete dysfunction in which there is a barrier to fertilization at the level of the acrosome reaction, zona pellucida binding or interaction, zona penetration, or fusion with the oolemma. ICSI is always indicated for patients who have unexplained failure of fertilization in two or more IVF-ET cycles.
2. Severe oligospermia can be treated with ICSI; if as many normal vital sperm can be recovered as there are oocytes to be inseminated, fertilization can be achieved in approximately 90% of these patients. In extreme cases of crypto-

zoospermia, where no sperm cells can be seen by standard microscopy, centrifugation of the neat sample at a higher than usual centrifugal force (1800 g, 5 minutes) may result in the recovery of an adequate number of sperm cells.
3. Severe asthenozoospermia, including patients with sperm ultrastructural abnormalities such as Kartagener's syndrome, or '9+0' axoneme disorders can be treated by ICSI.
4. Teratozoospermia, including absolute teratozoospermia or globozoospermia.
5. MESA (microsurgical epididymal sperm aspiration) and TESA (testicular biopsy extracted sperm) can be used to retrieve sperm for ICSI in patients with conditions such as congenital bilateral absence of the vas deferens or untreatable post-inflammatory obstruction of the vas.
6. With ejaculatory dysfunction, such as retrograde ejaculation – a sufficient number of sperm cells can usually be recovered from the urine.
7. Paraplegic males have been given the chance of biological fatherhood using electroejaculation and IVF; they may also be successfully treated using a combination of TESE and ICSI.
8. Immunological factors – couples in whom there may be antisperm antibodies in female sera / follicular fluid, or antisperm antibodies in seminal plasma following vasectomy reversal or genital tract infection can be sucessfully treated by ICSI.
9. Oncology – male patients starting chemotherapy or radiotherapy should have semen samples frozen for use in the future. Although the sperm quality of the frozen-thawed sperm may be grossly impaired, ICSI offers the patient an excellent chance of eventually achieving fertilization.

At the Lister Hospital (Chelsea Bridge Road, London SW1 8RH), the team led by Mr Hossam Abdulla and Mr Terry Leonard analysed their results of treatment of male factor infertility, comparing the pregnancy rates achieved after gamete intrafallopian transfer (GIFT), standard IVF, and ICSI. This analysis suggests the following indications for treatment, based upon parameters of semen assessment:

	ICSI	*Standard IVF*
Total sperm count	$<1\times10^6$ per ml	$>5\times10^6$ per ml
Motility	$<20\%$	$>30\%$
Progression	<1	>2
Motile concentration	$<100\,000$ per ml	$>5\times10^6$ per ml
Normal Motile Conc.	$<100\,000$ per ml	$>5\times10^6$ per ml

They suggest that cases with the following semen parameters should have either a trial of standard IVF first, or treatment in which the eggs are divided 50:50 for IVF and ICSI.

Total sperm count	Between 1 and 5×10^6
Motility	20–30%
Progression	1.5–2.0
Motile concentration	100 000 to 5×10^6
Normal motile concentration	100 000 to 5×10^6

ICSI now has a confirmed place not only in the treatment of male factor infertility, but also in cases of idiopathic infertility where the barrier to fertilization may include factors in the female partner which affect or involve the oocyte. To date published fertilization rates for most categories of patients reach 67%, with a clinical pregnancy rate of 36% and an ongoing/delivery rate of 28%.

Practical aspects

When scheduling patients for ICSI, unless the laboratory is fortunate in having a scientist dedicated entirely to carrying out each ICSI procedure, it is important that the whole IVF team should appreciate the extra dimension of time and effort which every case involves, and make an effort to schedule the entire laboratory workload accordingly. ICSI requires the same meticulous attention to detail required in all IVF manipulations, but the number of details requiring attention is dramatically increased. Successful results with ICSI can only be achieved with the dedication of concentrated time, effort, and patience.

Important considerations regarding the location of micromanipulation facilities

The laboratory should be on a ground floor, near a structural frame or wall to minimize vibration interference, and must be kept dust-free. The equipment must be installed on a substantial bench top, away from traffic of people or trolleys, etc. Subdued lighting is helpful for microscopy.

Well in advance of any ICSI procedure, ensure that the microscope is set up optically and checked. Ensure that the tool holders and entire micromanipulator system is correctly fitted and adjusted for optimal range of movement, and that the microtools can be accurately aligned.

Microtools

ICSI involves the use of two types of microtools: the holding pipette (a blunt-ended tube with constricted lumen) which is used to hold and immobilize the oocyte, and the injection pipette which will be used to aspirate and inject the sperm cell. Injection pipettes (of different diameters) may also be used to aspirate anucleate fragments, or for blastomere biopsy prior to pre-implantation diagnosis. A third type of microtool may be used for piercing or cutting the zona pellucida in assisted zona hatching techniques or partial zona drilling.

Specifically tooled, sterile, ready-to-use holding and injection pipettes are now commercially available from several different companies (COOK IVF, Swemed, Rochford Medical). For groups who are initiating an ICSI programme, ready-made pipettes provide a means of bypassing significant capital expenditure in obtaining equipment for their manufacture, and overcoming the hurdle of dedicating personnel and time to acquire the expertise involved in making them proficiently.

PVP preparation

Dissolve 1 g PVP-K90 (molecular weight 360 000 ICN Flow) in 10 ml culture grade water.
Dialyse the solution at 4 °C versus culture grade water for 2 days, changing the water seven times each day.
Dialysis tubing = Visking size 9–36/32″ (Medicell International Ltd, London, UK)
Lyophilise the dialysate, and store at room temperature until further use.
PVP (polyvinyl pyrrolidone) stock solution: 1 g lyophilised PVP dissolved in 10 ml HEPES buffered culture medium containing 0.5% bovine serum albumin. Filter through an 8 μm Millipore filter, and store at 4 °C for a maximum of 3 weeks.

Oocyte preparation and handling

Patients for ICSI have a scheduled oocyte retrieval after programmed superovulation, according to protocols described previously (see Preparation for oocyte retrieval, Chapter 2).

Oocyte identification is carried out immediately after follicle aspiration, using a dissecting microscope with heated stage. Take care to maintain stable temperature and pH of the aspirates at all times. At the end of the oocyte retrieval, note quality and maturity assessment of the oocytes, and then pre-incubate them for approximately 3 hours at 37 °C in an atmosphere of 5% CO_2 in air .

Preparation for injection: cumulus-corona removal

1. Hyaluronidase solution, 80 IU/ml: dissolve 1 mg of Hyalase (Type VIII, Sigma, cat. no. H3757) in 4 ml protein-free Earles balanced salt solution

(EBS), filter, and warm to 37°C. Prepare the hyaluronidase solution fresh daily, at least 1 hour before use.
2. Prepare a culture dish containing one drop of Hyalase solution and 5 wash drops of culture medium, covered with an overlay of equilibrated mineral oil. Incubate at 37 °C in the CO_2 incubator for 30–60 minutes.
3. Prepare a thin glass probe and some hand-drawn and fire-polished Pasteur pipettes, with the lumen ranging down to approximately 200 μm.
4. Remove the oocyte and hyalase dishes from the incubator, group the oocytes together in small batches (4–8 eggs per drop) and then wash the groups of oocytes through the hyalase drop, agitating gently until the cells start to dissociate (approximately 1 minute). Carefully aspirate the oocytes, leaving as much cumulus as possible behind. Wash by transferring them through at least 5 drops of culture medium, and change to a fine-bore pipette for aspiration in order to finally remove all of the coronal cells. All corona cells must be removed, as they will hinder the injection process by blocking the needle or obscuring clear observation of the cytoplasm and sperm.
5. Assess the quality and maturity of each oocyte under an inverted microscope. Use the glass probe to roll the oocytes around gently in order to identify the polar body, and examine the ooplasm for vacuoles or other abnormalities. Separate metaphase I or germinal vesicle (GV) oocytes from metaphase II oocytes, and label them.
6. Culture the dissected oocytes for a minimum of 1 hour before beginning micromanipulation.
7. Examine the oocytes again before starting the injection procedure to see if any more have extruded the first polar body. ICSI is carried out on all morphologically intact oocytes which have extruded the first polar body (Figure 12.1).

Preparation for injection

Injection dish

Materials: HEPES-buffered culture medium containing 0.5% BSA

10% PVP solution
Equilibrated paraffin oil
Shallow Falcon dish (type 1006)

1. Prepare the dish by pipetting eight small (2–5 μl) droplets of HEPES-buffered culture medium in a circle, and a ninth droplet containing PVP solution in the centre. These droplets must be positioned so that they are not too close to the central drop (to avoid mixing with the sperm/PVP) and not too close to the edge, where manipulation will be difficult. Number the droplets, and draw a circle on the bottom of the dish around the central droplet to facilitate rapid identification. Cover the drops with paraffin oil, warm the dish in the CO_2

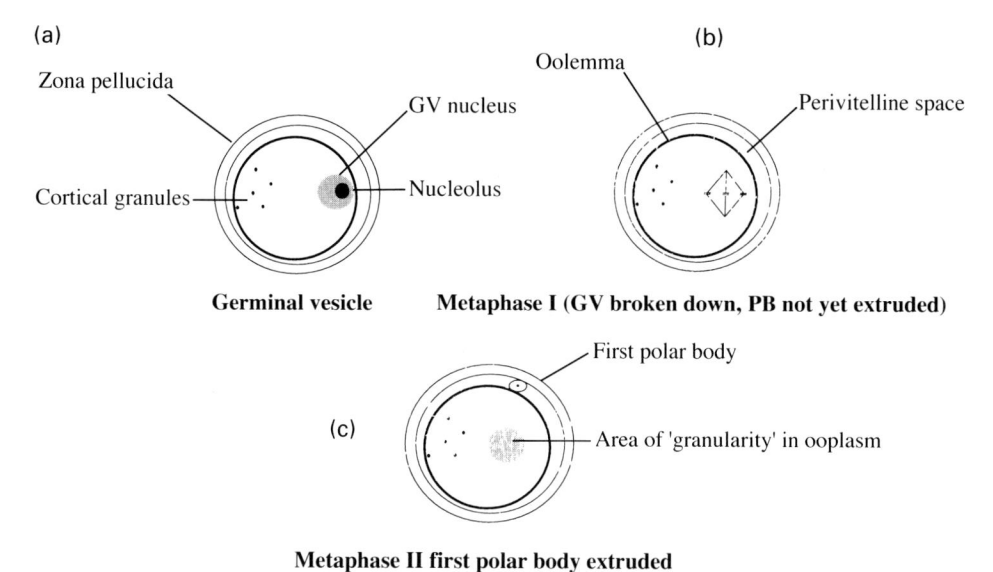

Figure 12.1 Variations in egg maturity found after hyalase treatment and corona dissection. (a) Germinal vesicle; (b) metaphase I; (c) metaphase II.

incubator for 20–30 minutes, and keep the dishes in the incubator until you are ready to begin.
2. At the same time, prepare and equilibrate another culture dish into which the oocytes will be transferred after injection.

Micromanipulator

1. Make sure that the heating stage on the microscope is warm, ensure that all controls can be comfortably operated, and that you are confident that all parts function smoothly before you begin. It is essential to check that you can smoothly carry out very small movements. This involves not only the equipment itself, but its position on the bench in relation to your (comfortable) seating position.
2. Insert holding and injection pipettes into the pipette holders, tighten well, and make sure (again) that there are no air bubbles in the tubing system. Bubbles interfere with accuracy when attempting to control movement with fine precision.
3. Align the pipettes so that the working tips are parallel to the microscope stage. First align the holding pipette under low magnification, then again under low magnification align the injection pipette. Check the position of both under high magnification. It is important to begin with pipettes in accurate alignment, with both working tips sharply in focus. If a part of the length is out of focus, the pipette is probably not parallel to the stage, but pointing upwards.
4. Adjust the injection controls: oil should just reach the distal end of the pipette;

do not try to fill the needle with oil, it won't work! Briefly touch the tips of both pipettes in oil, and then in medium, so that the ends fill by capillary action (a drop of oil behind the drop of medium will act as a buffer). The injection dish is still in the incubator, so you should be using a 'blank' dish for this!

Transfer the gametes to the injection dish

1. Slowly add a small aliquot of sperm suspension (0.3–5 µl, depending on the concentration of prepared sperm) to the edge of the central PVP droplet. The viscous solution should facilitate sperm handling by slowing down their motility, and also prevents the sperm cells from sticking to the injection pipette during the procedure. Be careful of sperm density: too many sperm will make sperm selection and immobilization more difficult.
2. After the sperm droplet has been carefully examined for the presence of debris or any other factors that might cause technical difficulties, examine all the denuded oocytes again for the presence of a first polar body; wash them with HEPES-buffered medium and transfer one oocyte into each oocyte droplet on the injection dish.
   Keep the oocytes in the incubator until you are confident that the injection procedure can proceed smoothly. Until sufficient experience of the procedure has been gained, it may be advisable to keep sperm and egg dishes separate, avoiding over-exposure of the oocytes while selecting and immobilizing sperm.
3. Place the injection dish with central sperm droplet on the microscope stage. Using the coarse controls of the manipulator, lower the injection pipette into the drop.

Sperm selection and immobilization

1. Try to select sperm which appear morphologically normal.
2. Motile spermatozoa are immobilized by crushing their tails: select the sperm to be aspirated, and lower the tip of the injection needle onto the midpiece of the sperm, striking down and across, and crushing the tail against the bottom of the dish. This 'tail crushing' impairs motility, and destabilizes the cell membrane; the latter may be required for sperm head decondensation. If the resulting sperm has a 'bent' tail, it will be difficult to aspirate into the needle, and will stick inside the needle. When this happens, the sperm must be abandoned and the procedure repeated with another sperm. Do not strike too hard, or the sperm will stick to the bottom of the dish, also making aspiration into the needle difficult. After some practice, sperm immobilization in routine ICSI cases can be carried out quite quickly. If the preparation contains only a few sperm with barely recognizable movement and a large amount of debris, this part of the procedure can be very tedious and require great patience!

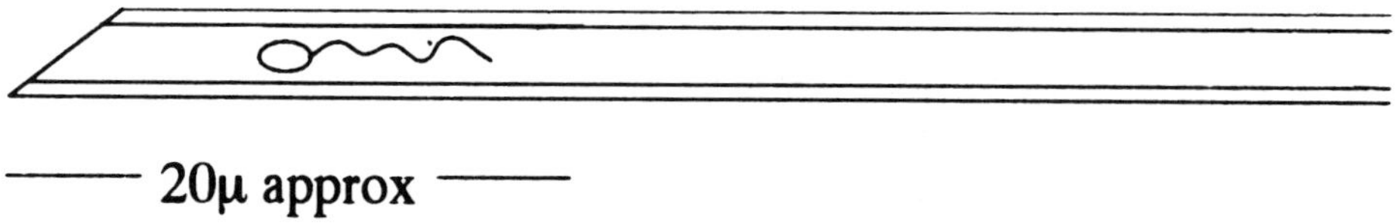

Figure 12.2 Single sperm inside microinjection needle prior to injection.

3. Aspirate the selected immobilized sperm, tail first, into the injection pipette. Position it approximately 20 µm from the tip (Figure 12.2).
4. Lift the injection needle slightly, and move the microscope stage so that the injection pipette is positioned in the first oocyte drop. If the sperm moves up the pipette (due to the difference in density between culture medium and PVP) bring it back near the tip before beginning the injection procedure.

Injection procedure

1. Lower the holding pipette into the first oocyte droplet, and position it adjacent to the cell. Using both microtools, slowly rotate the oocyte to locate the polar body and identify an area of apparent granularity (presumed to be the site of germinal vesicle breakdown, and should be avoided during injection). Aspirate gently so that the cell attaches to the pipette. The pressure should be great enough to hold the oocyte in place, but not so strong that it causes the oolemma to bulge outwards.
   Position the oocyte so that the polar body is at 6 or 12 o'clock, to minimize the possibility of damaging the meiotic spindle.
2. Move the injection pipette close to the oocyte, and check that it is in the same plane in apposition with the right outer border of the oolemma on the equatorial plane at the 3 o'clock position. Check that the sperm can be moved smoothly within the injection needle, and position it near the bevelled tip.
3. Advance the pipette until it penetrates the zona, and advance further through the ooplasm until the needle tip almost touches the 9 o'clock position. If the pipette is in the wrong plane, entry into the cell will be difficult. A break in the membrane must be seen, and this often requires negative pressure, sucking the membrane into the pipette before expelling the sperm. When it breaks, there will be a sudden acceleration of movement as cytoplasm and the spermatozoon will flow into the pipette. Inject the sperm slowly into the oocyte with a minimal amount of fluid (1–2 picolitres).
   The sperm should be ejected past the tip of the pipette, to ensure a tight insertion among the organelles which will hold it in place while the pipette is withdrawn. Some surplus medium may be re-aspirated to reduce the size of the breach created during perforation. If the ooplasm is elastic and difficult to break, it may be necessary to withdraw the pipette from the first membrane

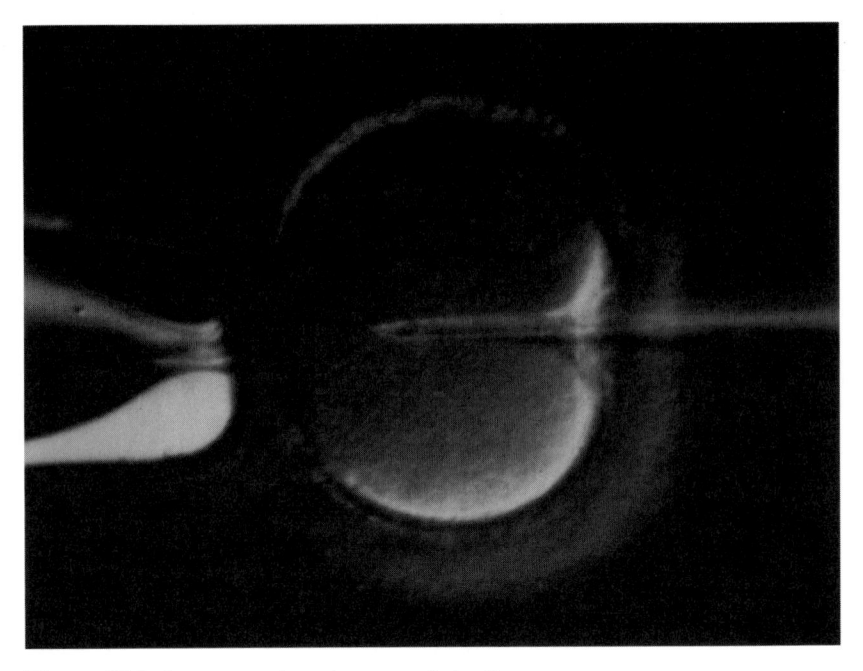

Figure 12.3 Intracytoplasmic sperm injection.

invagination and slowly repeat the procedure. Occasionally the sperm follows the pipette out, and may be released into the perivitelline space instead of the ooplasm (Figure 12.3).

4. Gently remove the injection pipette, and examine the breach area. The border of the opening should have a funnel shape, pointing in towards the egg. If the border of the oolemma is everted, cytoplasm may leak out, and the egg may subsequently degenerate. Release the oocyte from the holding pipette.
5. Repeat the sperm aspiration and injection until all the selected metaphase II oocytes have been injected.
6. Wash all the oocytes in culture medium, transfer to the prepared, warmed culture dish, and incubate overnight in the CO_2 incubator.

Injection procedure: important points!!!

1. All conditions must be stable: temperature, pH, equipment properly set up, adjusted, aligned, and checked for leaks and air bubbles. Check everything, including secure and comfortable operating position, before you begin.
2. Correct immobilization of sperm.
3. Advance far enough into the ooplasm with the injection pipette.
4. Ensure that the plasma membrane is broken.
5. Inject a minimal volume.
6. If the sperm comes out of the ooplasm into the perivitelline space, re-inject.

Intracytoplasmic sperm injection

(a) Nucleoli

2PN, 2nd PB
monospermic fertilization

(b)

3PN, 1st PB
monospermic digynic

(c)

Single pronucleus, 1 or 2 PB
?activated
(check again later)

(e)

Early cleavage

(d)

0 pronuclei, 1st PB
unfertilized

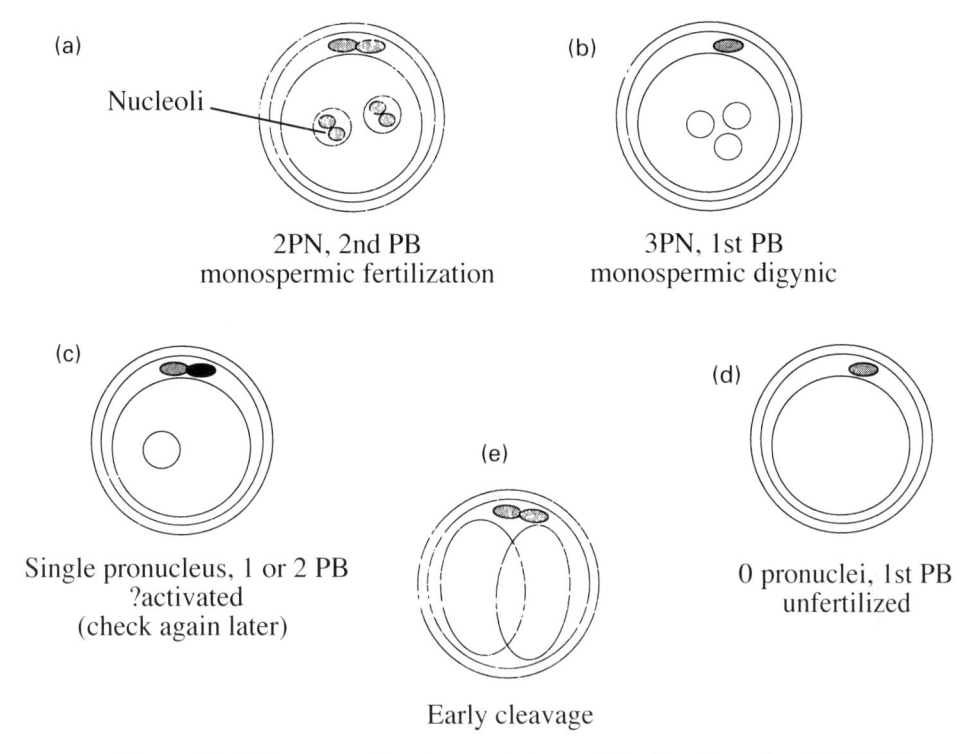

Figure 12.4 Diagrams showing variations of fertilization after ICSI. PN: pronuclei; PB: polar body. (a) Two pronuclei, 2 polar bodies; (b) three pronuclei, one polar body; (c) one pronucleus, two polar bodies; (d) No pronuclei, one polar body; (e) early cleavage.

Assessment of fertilization and cleavage

Sixteen to 18 hours after injection, assess the number and morphology of pronuclei several times through an inverted microscope, rolling the oocyte gently with a glass probe. Polar bodies should also be counted, with reference to digynic zygotes or activated eggs; polar bodies may fragment, even in normal monospermic fertilization. Rapid cleavage (20–26 hours post-injection) can occur in ICSI zygotes.

Evaluate normally fertilized, cleaved embryos after a further 24 hours of culture. Embryo transfer is usually performed approximately 48 hours after microinjection. Suitable supernumerary embryos may be cryopreserved either on day 1 (pronucleate stage) or on day 2 (early cleavage stage) (Figure 12.4).

No fertilization after ICSI

Complete failure of fertilization is rare after ICSI; most of these cases involve semen containing no motile sperm, or round-headed sperm. Some cases of failed fertilization may be attributed to low oocyte number, abnormal morphological appearance, or fragile oocytes which are easily damaged after ICSI.

Transport ICSI

In the same manner that a central IVF laboratory can be utilized to offer assisted conception treatment at nearby peripheral hospitals or clinics, a central ICSI laboratory can offer this specialized technique to peripheral hospitals which do not have the equipment or expertise. Pre-ovulatory oocytes and prepared sperm from patients are transported from the peripheral unit by the male partner immediately after the oocyte recovery procedure. Culture tubes containing the gametes are transported in a portable incubator, as described for transport IVF. On arrival at the central unit, the oocytes can be transferred to culture dishes and prepared for the ICSI procedure, and sperm preparation assessed and adjusted if necessary. Fertilized oocytes are cultured to the early cleavage stage, and the embryos may then be transported by the male partner back to the peripheral unit for the embryo transfer procedure. Supernumerary embryos may also be cryopreserved at the central unit if appropriate.

As with transport IVF, cooperation between participating units is particularly important in order to provide an effective service. Well planned protocols are essential for selection, consultation, and counselling of patients, the handling, preparation and transport of gametes, and communication of treatment cycle details/transport arrangements between units.

Equipment for ICSI

For microinjection

Dissecting microscope with heated stage
Inverted microscope with heated stage, attached to micromanipulators
    $4 \times$ objective for locating eggs and drops
    $20 \times$ objective for microsurgery
    $15 \times$ eyepiece
    Hoffman modulation or Nomarski optics
    Video monitoring facility
Bilateral micromanipulators for manipulation in three dimensions
Microtool holders
Two suction devices with steel syringes (80–100 µl) filled with light mineral oil (BDH), or appropriate alternative device for controlling holding and injection micropipettes
Incubator
Supply of 5% CO_2 in air

For making microtools

Borosilicate glass capillary tubing
Micropipette puller
Power supply with controlled variable voltage
Power cleaner to overcome power surges in mains electricity
Microforge
Microbeveller
Oven for heat sterilization

Supplies

Shallow Falcon petri dishes (Type 1006)
Culture medium
Culture medium + HEPES
Bovine serum albumin (BSA)
Hyaluronidase solution
Mineral oil
PVP solution
Pasteur pipettes
Hand-pulled polished glass pipettes
Pipette bulbs
Holding pipettes
ICSI needles

Adjustment of Narishige manipulators for ICSI (with thanks to Terry Leonard)

This guide refers to Nikon/Narishige system; the same principles apply to an Olympus system, but the details are slightly different.

Before attempting to fit or adjust the micromanipulators, first adjust the microscope optically, ideally using an oocyte in the same type of petri dish to be used for ICSI. The microscope settings will influence the working distance of the microtools. The final position of the micromanipulators on the microscope will depend upon:

a) the angle at which the tool holder is fixed
b) the combined length of the tool holder and needle from the point where it is held in the tool holder attachment to the centre of the light source.

Before finding the ideal position for the micromanipulators, they should be fitted correctly to the microscope, and final adjustments made later.

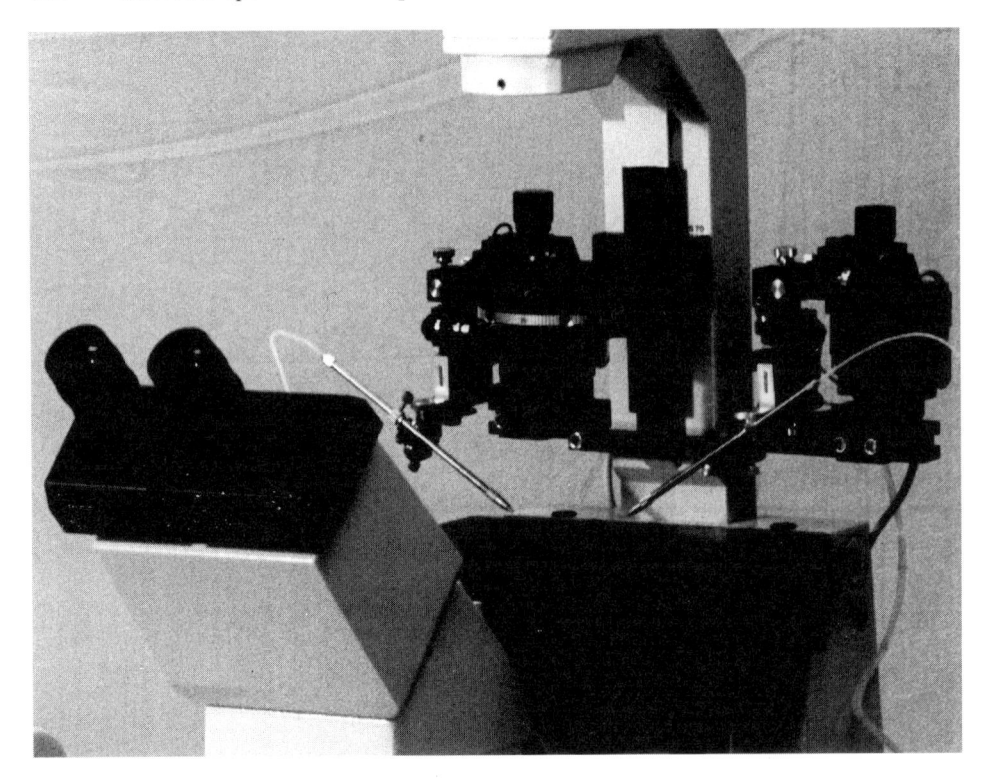

Figure 12.5 Nikon/Narishige coarse manipulator mounting.

Micromanipulator parts

1. Mounting bar: this joins the coarse manipulator to the microscope.
2. Coarse manipulator: consists of three parts, each controlling one of the three dimensions of movement. There are two types: manually operated and motor driven.
3. Fine manipulator: consists of two parts:
    a) the driving section: attached to the coarse manipulator, controls fine movements directed by the joystick.
    b) ball joint/tool holder attachment: attached to the driving section, used both to hold the microtool holder and to vary the angle at which it is held.
4. Joystick: links to the driving section via oil-filled tubes. The movement of the joystick is scaled down and transferred to the fine manipulator.

The mounting arrangement which attaches the coarse manipulator to the microscope is L-shaped. In the Nikon/Narishige system, the mounting is fitted to the illumination pillar as illustrated in Figure 12.5.

The mounting bar position is marked with a white L-shape.

The mounting bars have tracks into which the coarse manipulator fits, and

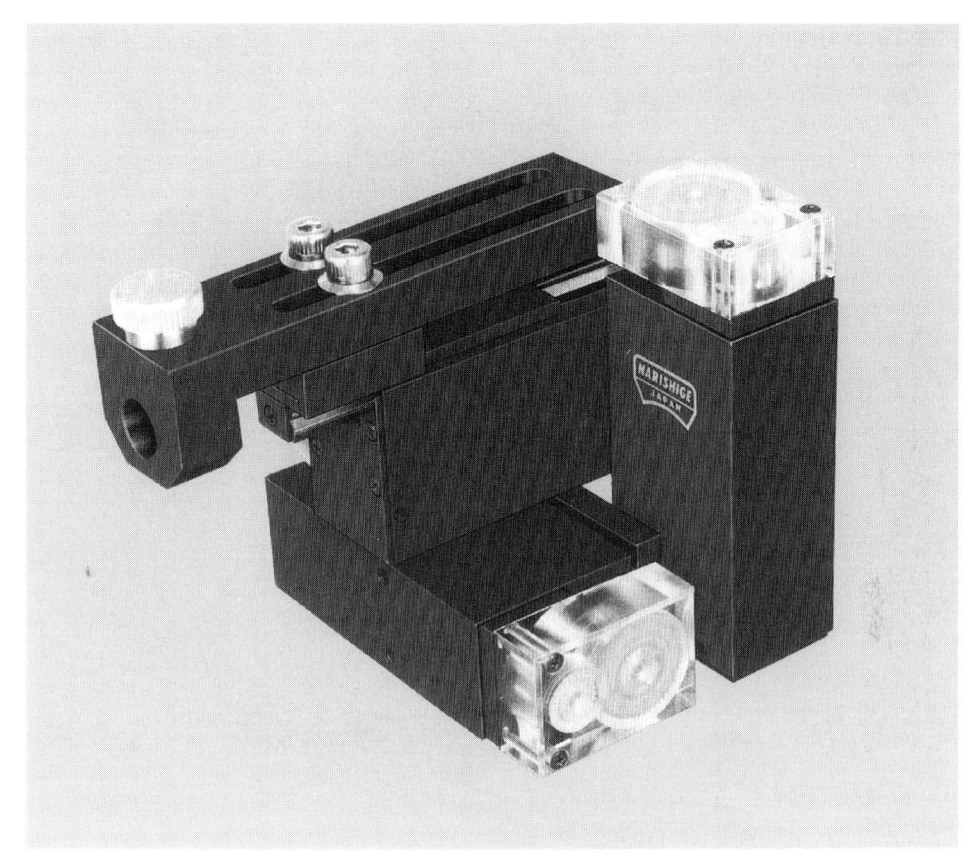

Figure 12.6 Adjusting the coarse manipulator.

the position of the coarse manipulator can be adjusted along these tracks. The entire mounting bar can be adjusted up and down.

Adjusting the coarse manipulators

1. Set the mounting bars at 90 degrees from the microscope stage or bench top.
2. Set the second part of the mounting at 90 degrees to the first, and ensure that the track is set flat.
3. Attach the coarse micromanipulator and adjust the lower section (left/right movement) so that it is parallel with the mounting bar. Set the other two sections of the coarse manipulator at right angles to each other (Figure 12.6).

Attaching the fine manipulator

The fine manipulator is attached to the coarse manipulator by a small metal rod (coupling bar). This can be screwed into one of the two holes on the driving section of the fine manipulator, depending on the side on which it is to be used.

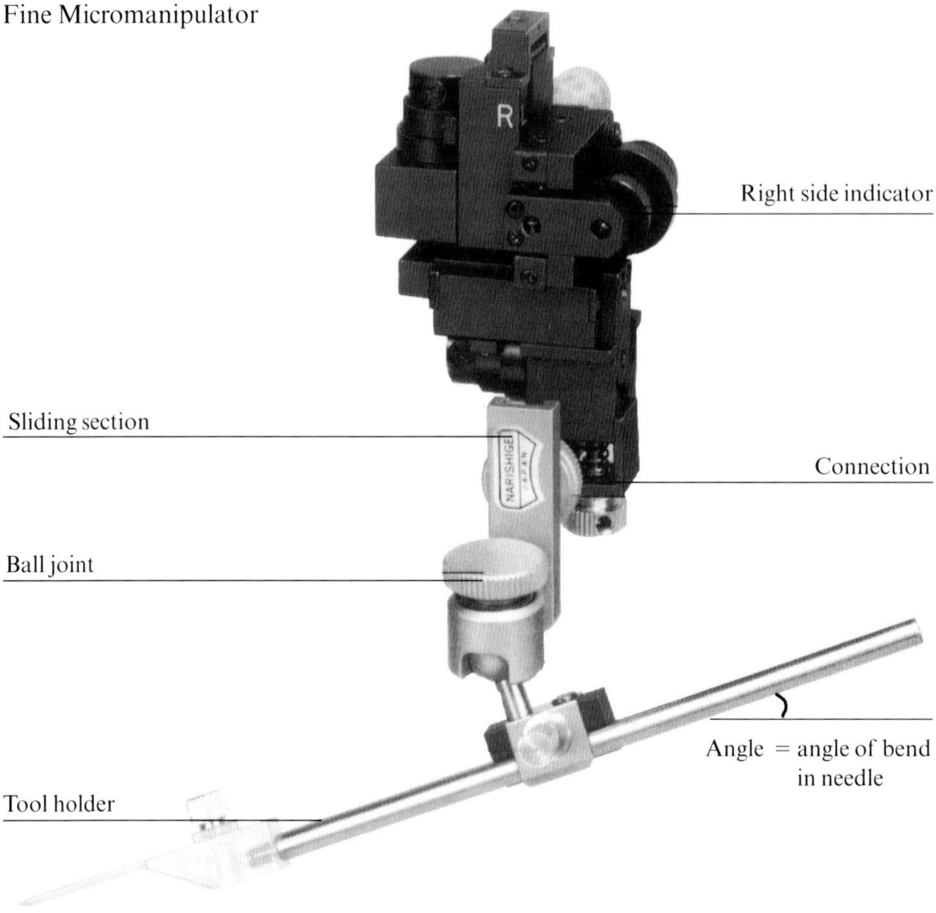
Fine Micromanipulator
R
Right side indicator
Sliding section
NARISHIGE JAPAN
Connection
Ball joint
Angle = angle of bend in needle
Tool holder

Figure 12.7 Attaching the fine manipulator.

In order to fit the fine manipulator on the right hand side, find the 'R' mark on the driving section and screw the coupling bar into the hole directly behind this mark. Attach the coupling bar/driving section to the coarse manipulator and tighten. Position the driving section so that it is parallel with the microscope or 90 degrees to the bench. Attach the left hand side in the same manner, screwing the coupling bar into the hole directly behind the 'L' mark. Arrange the joy-sticks so that the 'R' and 'L' marks are facing the operator on the appropriate sides (Figure 12.7).

Attaching the ball joint/tool holder attachment

The ball joint/tool holder attachment has a black metal bar projecting from it. This is fitted into the V-groove of the driving unit. The ball joint is then rotated to an appropriate angle so that when a needle is held in it, the tip of the microtool will be parallel with the microscope stage. The extent to which it is rotated will depend upon the angle at which the microtool is bent. For example, for a microtool which is angled at 35 degrees from the plane of the needle, the ball joint must be rotated 35 degrees anti-clockwise from the vertical position (Figure 12.7).

The manipulators should now be attached in the correct manner, but they may not be in the optimal working position. The ideal position will vary depending upon the angle of the needle and the combined length of the microtool and tool holder. It is therefore best to have a fixed tool angle, a fixed length of projection of the tool from the tool holder, and a fixed (marked) point where the tool holder is clamped to the tool holding attachment. If any of these three factors change, the fine adjustments will require re-setting.

Finding the best position for the micromanipulators

Adjust the three coarse manipulators so that they are in the middle of their range of movements.

Adjust the range of movements of the three fine manipulators on the joystick so that they are in the middle of the scales.

Forward/backward movement

First ensure that the hole in the stage is positioned directly in the middle of the light path. View the micromanipulator from the side of the microscope, then align the tool holder attachment with the middle of the hole in the microscope stage. This can be adjusted by changing the position of the coupling bar on the fine manipulator, the projection from the ball joint, or the two screws (Figure 12.6) on the very top of the coarse manipulator which controls the forward/backward movement.

Left/right movement

Place a microtool holder together with a microtool in the tool holder attachment. Attach it at the very tip of the tool holder, and gently slide it along towards the light source. If it will not reach the light source, the entire manipulator should be moved to the left. Likewise, if it reaches it too soon (before the marked point) the entire manipulator should be shifted to the right. This adjustment is performed by loosening the bolts which attach the coarse micromanipulator to the mounting bar. After this adjustment, ensure that the micromanipulator is still parallel to the bar.

Up/down movement

Adjust the manipulator so that the microtool is approximately 0.5 cm from the surface of the stage. For large adjustments loosen the bolts which attach the mounting bar to the microscope and move up or down. Remember to ensure that it is still 90 degrees from the bench after adjustment. Fine up/down adjustments can be made by moving the small sliding section above the ball joint.

Alignment of the ICSI needle in the manipulator

When using a Narishige tool holder, push the needle in so that 4–5 cm of the needle is outside the holder. Place the tool holder in the right hand micromanipulator with the needle tip over the light source. The angle at which the tool holder is held should be such that the angled tip of the needle is parallel with the stage of the microscope. Under a very low power ($\times 4$ objective), place the tip of the ICSI needle in the field of vision of the microscope. Loosen the tool holder attachment and rotate the tool holder so that the bent portion of the needle appears to be straight. Ensure that you can focus on a good portion of the needle (from the tip). The portion of the needle after the bend will be out of focus. If the microscope has a graticule, make sure that the movement of the needle from right to left does not vary. Place the ICSI needle along the middle of the microspcope field with the tip almost in the centre. Align the holding pipette in the same manner so that the tips of the needle and pipette are facing each other, and then raise them up away from the stage.

Perform the final adjustment of the angle at which the tool holder is held within a sperm droplet. Find a non-motile sperm and then bring the ICSI needle into the same optical plane. Raise the ICSI needle off the surface of the petri dish very slightly, move it over the top of the sperm, and try to touch the sperm by lowering the needle. If it is impossible to touch the sperm, the needle is not parallel with the surface. The end of the needle will be lower than the tip. To rectify this, raise the needle and rotate the ball joint anticlockwise slightly, lower the needle, and try to touch the sperm again. If the tip of the needle can touch the sperm, but the rest of the needle is not in focus, the tip of the needle is lower than the bend. To rectify this, raise the needle and rotate the ball joint slightly in a clockwise direction.

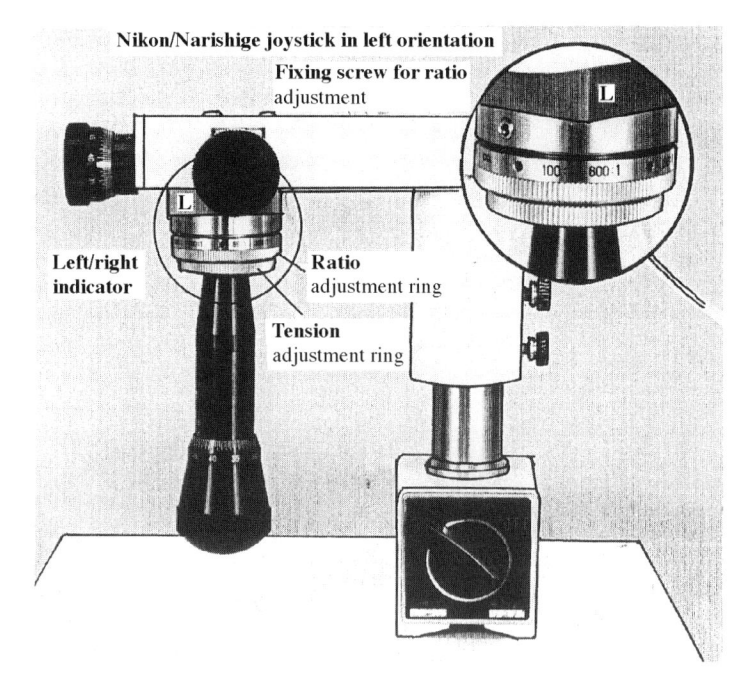

Figure 12.8 Arranging the joysticks.

Ratio of movement and joysticks

1. Focus on the tip of the microtool.
2. Loosen the two screws on the movement adjustment rings.
3. Ignore the ratios written on the side of the joystick, and rotate the adjustment rings anticlockwise until you are satisfied with the movement as observed down the microscope.

When all of the adjustments and alignments are made, the need to repeat any of these should be minimal, unless the style of the needle or tool holder is changed. When removing the tool holder from its attachment, keep the ball joint at the same angle so that when a new needle is inserted, it will be at approximately the right angle for use. Fine adjustments will be necessary for each manipulation (Figure 12.8).

168 *Micromanipulation techniques*

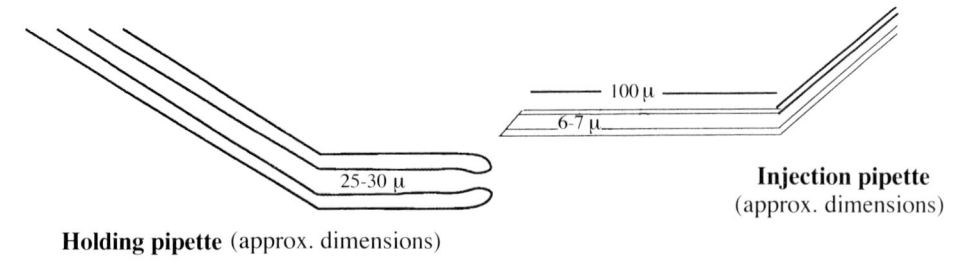

Figure 12.9 Injection and holding pipettes.

Microtool preparation

The following details describe the procedures currently in use at Bourn Hall, and are intended as guidelines for reference only. Specific details will vary according to individual equipment, facilities, and the personnel using them, and a significant amount of 'trial and error' adjustment is to be expected.

Equipment

Microtools are made by applying heat and force to capillary tubing. The heat source is a filament controlled by voltage applied through an electrical resistance device and, when the glass is semi-melted, force is provided by a simple spring pulling device with adjustable settings. The tools can then be modified using a grinding wheel to grind the tip to the required size, and a microforge to cut, bend, constrict or pull the tapered sections of the micropipette.

Capillary tubing

Most microtool holders on micromanipulation equipment are designed for tubing of a specific diameter, commonly 1 mm. Tubing is available in a variety of wall thicknesses: a thin wall helps to maintain a large lumen with the smallest tip diameter possible, whereas thicker walled tubing is better for holding pipettes.

We use borosilicate glass capillary tubing, from Clark Electromedical, supplied in containers of 500 pieces.

       For holding pipettes: 1 mm × 0.78 mm (outer/inner diameter), 100 mm length (GC100–10)
       Injection pipettes: 1 mm30 × 0.58 mm, 100 mm length (GC100T-10)
(See Figure 12.9).

PCP7 Plug board (Research Instruments)

Used to supply a controlled voltage which heats the pipette puller and microforge filaments. The amp-meter readings should be set before starting and, because mains electricity varies in different locations, suggested peg settings are approximate only.

IMMAC power cleaner

Used to stabilize the power supply to overcome power surges in mains electricity.

Micropipette puller (MPP11, Research Instruments)

Can be used to draw any type of pipette, to a range of diameters. The adjustable controls allow repeatable control over the pulling process by adjusting distance travelled with the left and right carriage stops and force of pull with the adjustable spring force. Time is varied manually by using a stopwatch to time the operation of the carriage release pin .

More sophisticated pullers (e.g. Sachs-Flaming puller, Sutter Instruments) are available, which incorporate microprocessor control over the variable parameters. Programmes for particular tools can be entered into the machine and stored in memory slots.

Microforge (Research Instruments)

Used to alter the pulled section of the capillary: the tapered sections of a micropipette can be cut, bent, constricted, pulled, or polished. It consists of a heating filament and micromanipulators used to control the position of the microtool in relation to the filament. It also has a magnification system (80 ×) with an eyepiece micron scale arranged to focus on the filament and micropipette during forging procedures. The temperature of the filament is controlled by the same plug board used for the puller.

Microbeveller or microgrinder (Research Instruments)

Used for adjusting the size of the bevel on injection pipettes. It has a 20 × eyepiece incorporating 100XY graticule and 20 × objective. Each small division of the graticule = 3.5 µm approximately.

The abrasive grinding wheel is partially immersed in a water bath, and the wheel gradually grinds the tip of the pipette to the appropriate size. The pipette is observed through the eyepiece at 1–2 minute intervals, until the required dimensions are reached.

Pipette storage containers

Pipettes may be safely stored by immobilizing them with Blu-tack inside plastic petri dishes. Glass storage containers with Pyrex glass covers (Research Instruments) are used for heat sterilization.

Oven for heat sterilization

Glassware and pipettes are heat sterilized at 180 °C for 2 hours.

Attention must also be paid to the environment for microtool preparation, and to allocating dedicated laboratory space and scientist time. Vibration will interfere with the necessary precision, and the individual units may be isolated on foam pads if necessary. Adequate lighting is very important, and the microforge should be in a position in which it can be comfortably operated. The environment should also be dust-free, free of drafts and the interruption of slamming doors, etc.

Procedure

Pulling

A pulled section of capillary tubing must be produced, which is at least 1 cm in length, and the correct diameter in the area of the tip. Different pipette shapes are obtained by different combinations of spring force, length of pull, and filament temperature, and different specifications of glass have different pulling characteristics, i.e. thick-walled (holding pipette) and thin-walled (injection pipette) tubing behave differently. For thick-walled tubing, the second pull is usually at a lower temperature than the first pull, and for thin-walled tubing the second pull often has to be at a higher temperature than the first pull. The settings listed here are specifically for ICSI pipettes, and are for guidance only. They may require adjustment according to variables such as air temperature, electricity supply, individual variation, etc. Pipettes for other uses such as zona cutting or drilling or blastomere biopsy require different settings and procedures.

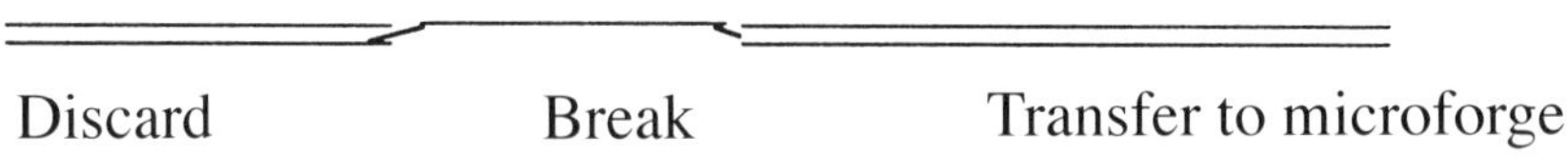

Discard   Break   Transfer to microforge

Figure 12.10 Breaking a capillary.

Holding pipettes

Use thick-walled tubing, 100 × 0.58, 100 mm length

Settings: Puller: Left carriage stop   75
                     Traverse   10
                     Right carriage stop   0
                     Force   6

Microtool preparation 171

Current (PCP7 power controller) at 6.5
(Top Red 6, Bottom Red 5)

1. 'Soak' (apply the current) for 15 seconds, release the traverse pin to effect the pull, and then switch off the current. Remove the tubing, the piece on the RIGHT side will be used; break the tubing manually near the end of the tapering (Figure 12.10).
2. Transfer the pulled pipette to the microforge. Move the pipette under the glass bead, positioned tangentially to the surface of the bead at the area where a break is required. Heat the bead at a low setting, until it appears just noticeably hot (Top Black 3, Bottom Black 5), and carefully bring the needle into contact with the bead. When the two surfaces adhere, immediately turn the filament off. The pipette should break cleanly as the bead cools. Jagged or angled breaks can be avoided by keeping the two surfaces as parallel as possible. Slight angles or imperfections in the break are irrelevant, as the final 'polishing' step will melt these down. If the tip has more substantial deviations, it will have to be rebroken, provided that it is possible to do so without losing the appropriate diameter.

Insert pipette into microforge holder

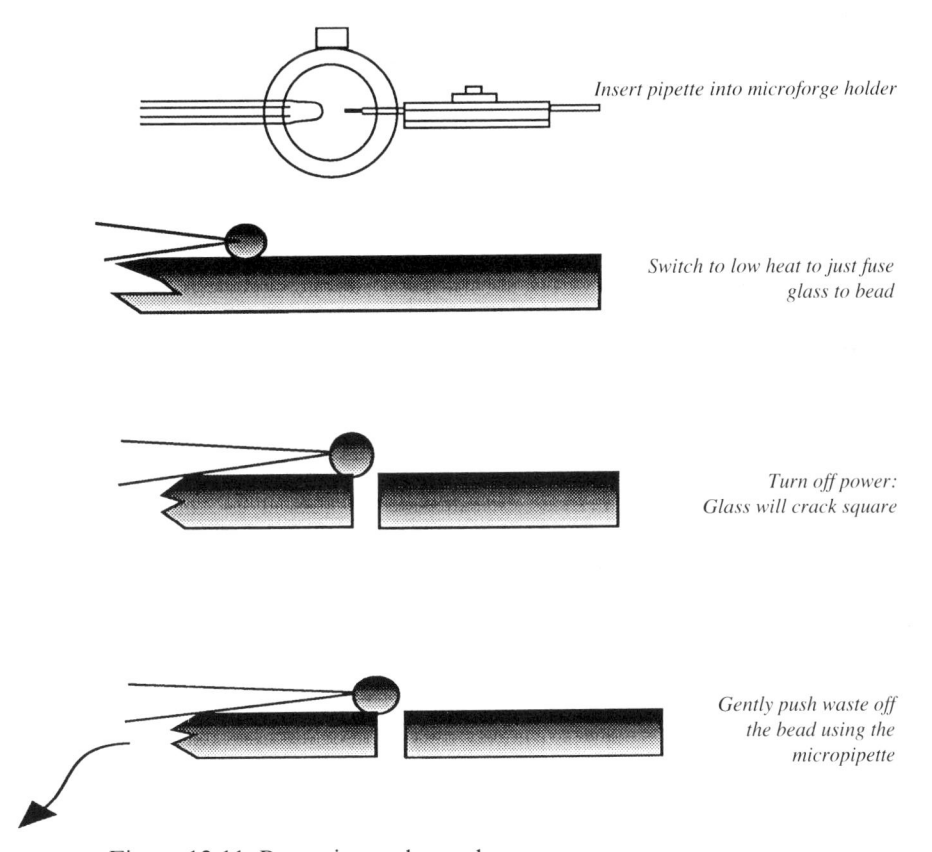

Switch to low heat to just fuse glass to bead

Turn off power: Glass will crack square

Gently push waste off the bead using the micropipette

Figure 12.11 Preparing a clean edge.

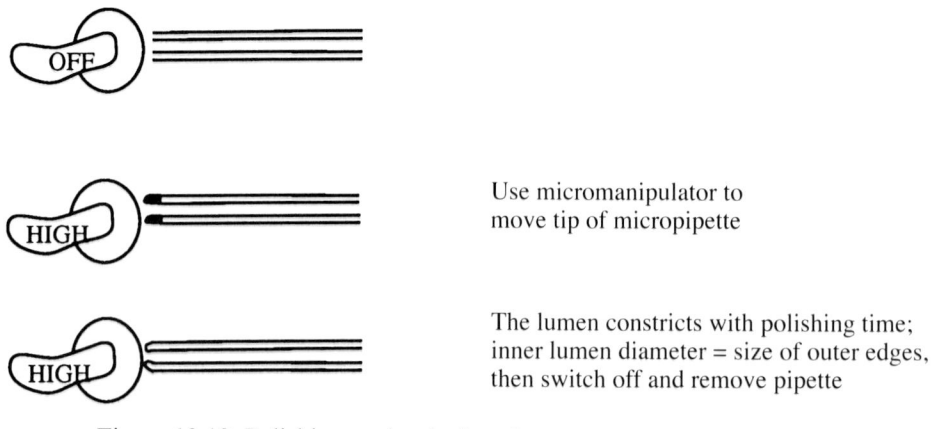

Figure 12.12 Polishing and reducing tip.

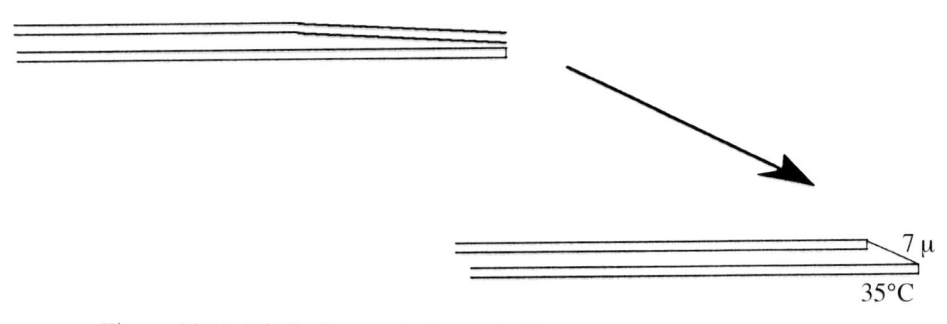

- OFF
- HIGH — Use micromanipulator to move tip of micropipette
- HIGH — The lumen constricts with polishing time; inner lumen diameter = size of outer edges, then switch off and remove pipette

Figure 12.13 Tip before and after grinding.

7 μ
35°C

Injection pipettes

The tips should be long, thin, and reasonably parallel, to minimize the size of the hole created in the zona and the oolemma. The holes must be small enough to avoid the injection of too much medium at the the time of injection, and to prevent loss of cytoplasm on needle withdrawal.

Use thin-walled tubing, 100 × 0.78, 100 mm length
Two separate pulls are required for each needle

1. Settings: Pull (1) Left carriage stop 55
   Current: 6.5
   (Top Red 6, Bottom Red 5)
   Traverse 10
   Right carriage stop 0
   Force 4

Insert the tubing, 'soak' for 10 seconds, then release the traverse pin. Switch off the current when the pull stops.

Microtool preparation

    Pull (2)   Left carriage stop   100
                 Traverse   0
                 Right carriage stop   10
                 Force   4
                 Current   6.5 (Red)

Switch on the current, release the pin (no 'soaking'), switch off the current when the pull stops.

Use the tubing on the LEFT side.

2. The beveller is then used to grind the end of the pipette so that the tip has an outer diameter of 7 μm (2 graticules on the scale) and an angle of approximately 35 degrees (Figure 12.13).

   Load the needle into the right hand groove of the holder, apply positive air pressure with a syringe, and grind with the wheel set at full speed. The grinding time will vary according to the initial tip size, and progress of the grinding should be regularly monitored accordingly (e.g. initial size 3–4 μm, grind for approximately 5 minutes, check every 1 or 2 minutes).

   Keeping the needle in the holder, check that the bevel is suitable, and then turn it so that the opening of the needle faces towards you. Mark the top of the pipette with a marker pen. The grinding wheel must be kept clean, by rubbing regularly with abrasive paper. The purified water in the water bath must also be replaced regularly.

3. Microforge: to add a bend, and modify the tip if necessary.

   Insert the needle into the holder so that the bevel is facing towards you, i.e. rotate the mark at the tip of the needle 90 degrees away from you.

   Heat the filament: Black Top 3, Bottom Black 5 (this must be adjusted by trial and error, so that it is neither too high nor too low!)

   Add a 30 degree bend: move the angle adjuster to the sixth division, and bring the needle towards the heated bead until the tip of the needle is horizontal; then switch the current off (Figure 12.14).

   If necessary, a spike or point can be added by gently fusing the tip of the needle to the heated bead (same setting as for making the 30 degree bend), and then pulling the needle away from the bead before switching the current off.

   NB: If the needle has a good bevel and sharp tip after adding the 30 degree angle, the last step, which can be very difficult, is not necessary.

4. Place carefully into glass pipette container, and heat sterilise at 180 °C for 2 hours.

Notes on pipette pulling

First Pull (injection pipette) *or Only Pull* (holding pipette)

174 *Micromanipulation techniques*

(a) Filament with glass bead

Move the angle adjuster to the sixth division

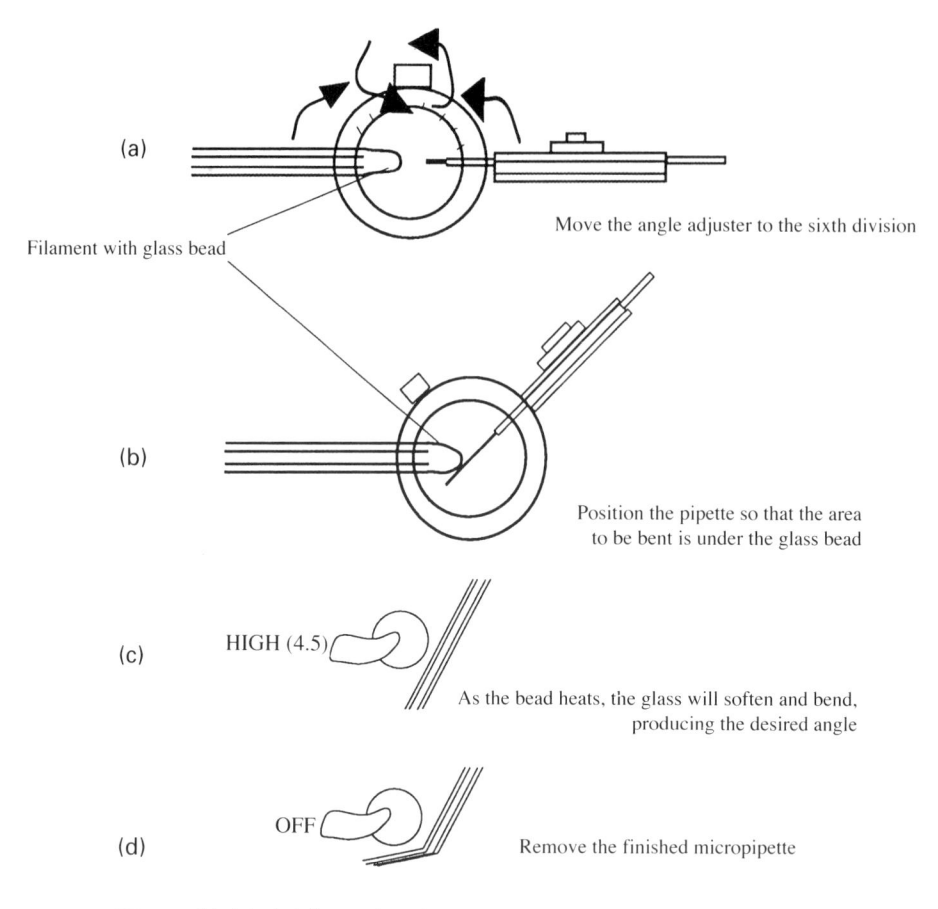

(b) Position the pipette so that the area to be bent is under the glass bead

(c) HIGH (4.5)

As the bead heats, the glass will soften and bend, producing the desired angle

(d) OFF

Remove the finished micropipette

Figure 12.14 Adding a bend.

Pipette too thin:

1. Move the carriage stop to make the pull shorter
2. Increase filament heat
3. Lower spring force by 0.5, 1.0 or 2.0 divisions

Pipette too thick:

1. Make pipette longer by moving the carriage stop
2. Lower the filament temperature by altering the power controller settings
3. Increase the spring force by 0.5 division or more if necessary

Second Pull

Pipette breaks before second pull (when moving the thin part back inside the filament coil):

1. Increase filament heat slightly on first pull (to make a slightly thicker pipette)

Microtool preparation

Pipette too thin:

1. Move carriage stop on the first pull, to create a shorter pull
2. Increase filament temperature slightly, by altering power controller settings on the first pull

Pipette too thick:

1. Move the carriage stop on the first pull to create a longer pull
2. Lower filament temperature slightly by altering the power controller settings on the first pull

Profile of the pipette is incorrect:

1. Alter the spring force, i.e.   First pull = 5, Second pull = 7, then try
    First pull = 5, Second pull = 6, or 6.5

Notes on the Microforge

Setting up

Insert a preformed filament of platinum-iridium wire into the filament holder. Using the micrometer stage, move the filament just to the left of the centre of the field of view. A new filament's heat response to the voltage applied may vary from the old filament, and changes to the filament such as glass ball size and even the surrounding air flow can affect the heat/voltage response. As the filament heats up, it will expand in size, and this expansion will vary between different filaments. Care must be taken to monitor this expansion, so that the hot filament is not driven directly into a needle during forging! During forging procedures it is usually best to heat the filament initially at a low voltage setting, increase as necessary.

Setting a glass bead onto the filament

Pull a sharp needle on the puller, and clamp it into position on the microforge with the tip facing the filament. Heat the filament so that the glass easily melts, and bring the needle tip into contact with the hot filament so that a bead of glass melts on the filament surface. Draw the needle away and turn the heat off; a glass bead should be left attached to the surface of the filament. This may require several steps of moving the needle into and away from the filament, until an appropriate size is reached; then heat the filament to round out the mass of glass. Once set up, a bead can be used for some time. When it eventually becomes too large or misshapen, it should be removed and renewed.

Cleaning glass from the filament

When the bead acquires too much adherent glass, the size can be reduced by heating the filament until it is dull orange in colour, and the rolling the tip of a waste pipette along the filament so glass from the filament adheres to the pipette. The section of tip used should have a diameter of approximately 70 μm.

Loading the micropipette

Clamp the micropipette into the carriage by closing the lid between finger and thumb. With the lever of the XY-positioner in the vertical, and the rotator in the horizontal position, slide the pipette so that it can be conveniently visualised. Using the lever-micromanipulator, check that the tip can be moved to touch the filament, and leave it well clear of the filament. Lightly clamp the carriage on its bar.

Assisted hatching

Jacques Cohen postulates that an inability of blastocysts to hatch from the zona pellucida may be one of the factors involved in the high implantation failure rate of human IVF procedures. The human zona becomes more brittle and loses its elasticity after fertilization, and spontaneous hardening also occurs after in vitro culture and in vivo aging. It also changes in its receptivity to decreased pH (it is easier to create a hole with acid Tyrode's solution in a zygote than in an unfertilized oocyte).

Early observations from videocinematography studies suggested that embryos which show a thick, even zona pellucida on day 2 had a poor prognosis for implantation. In addition, embryos produced as a result of microsurgical fertilization had a higher implantation rate, and when cultured in vitro hatched one day earlier than expected (day 5 instead of day 6). Following these observations, a series of experiments in a mouse embryo system led to the development of a clinical protocol based upon the following results:

1. Large holes are more efficient in supporting hatching than small holes: if the hole is too small, the embryo can become 'trapped' and fail to hatch. Zona drilling using an acid Tyrode's solution prevented 'trapping' which occurred as a result of mechanical partial zona drilling, and optimal hole size is approximately half the size of a single blastomere: 15–20 μm.
2. Embryos with such large gaps in their zonae should be transferred after the onset of compaction, on day 3: if embryo transfer is traumatic, blastomeres may escape through the gap in the zona; embryo transfer must therefore be gentle and atraumatic.

3. The artifical gap in the zona may also allow invasion of toxins into the embryo, with immune cell invasion or release of cytotoxins from neighbouring non-invasive immune cells; therefore prophylactic steroid and antibiotic treatment is recommended after embryo transfer.
4. Embryos must be pre-selected for assisted hatching, based upon previous IVF history (repeated failed implantation), maternal age, basal FSH levels, cleavage rates and morphology of the embryos with attention to zona thickness or variation.

Protocol

(Adapted from J. Cohen (1992) Zona pellucida micromanipulation and consequences for embryonic development and implantation. *In Micromanipulation of Human Gametes and Embryos*, chapter 8, J. Cohen, H.F. Malter, B.E. Talansky, and J. Grifo, Raven Press, New York.)

1. Perform zona drilling with acid Tyrode's (AT) solution approximately 72 hours after oocyte retrieval, with embryo transfer 5 to 7 hours later (i.e. drill before the formation of intercellular connections, but transfer after they have been established).
2. Perform the procedure in HEPES-buffered human tubal fluid (HTF) medium with 15% serum.
3. Use a straight microtool with an aperture of 7–8 μm.
4. Use mouth-controlled suction for the zona drilling procedure.
5. Embryos are contained in small microdroplets (25 μl) under mineral oil in a depression slide or shallow Falcon 1006 dish containing one droplet of AT solution and four wash droplets.
6. Micromanipulate each embryo individually, and immediately wash each, one to four times to remove the acidic medium (Figure 12.15).

Tyrode's solution is acidified by titrating to pH 2.3–2.5 with HCl.

Step-by-step

1. Front load the microneedle before each micromanipulation, using mouth-controlled suction.
2. Clamp the embryo onto the holding pipette (syringe suction system) so that the acidic Tyrode's filled microneedle at the 3 o'clock area is exposed to empty perivitelline space or to extracellular fragments. There should be no more than a 2 second delay from the time the hatching needle enters the drop to the initiation of hatching.
3. Expel acidic medium gently over a small (30 μm) area by holding the needle tip very close to the zona. Small circular motions can avoid excess acid in a single area.

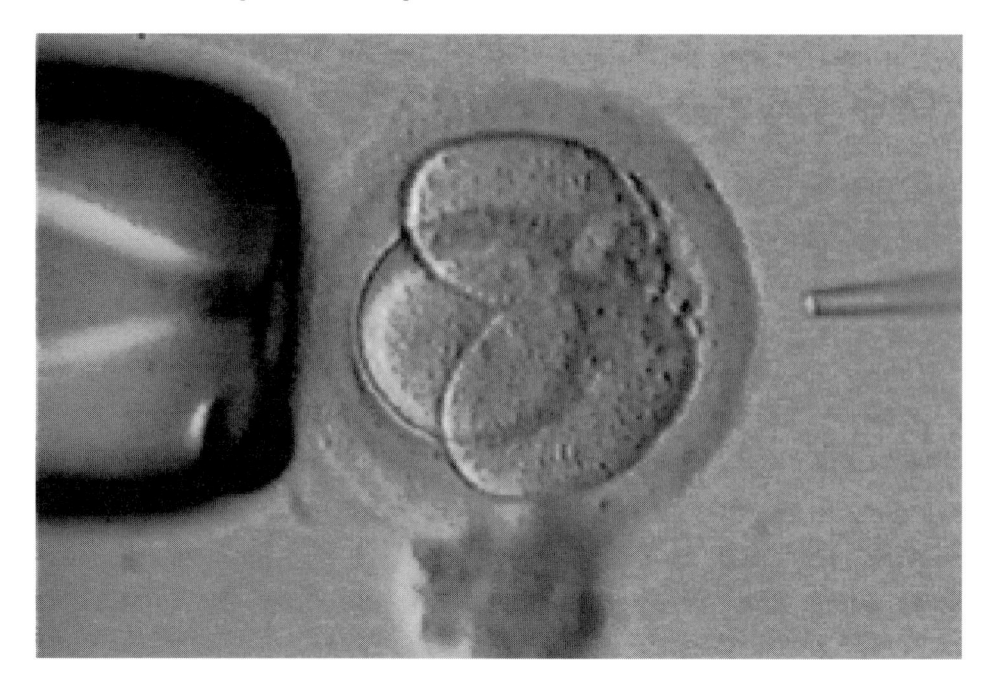

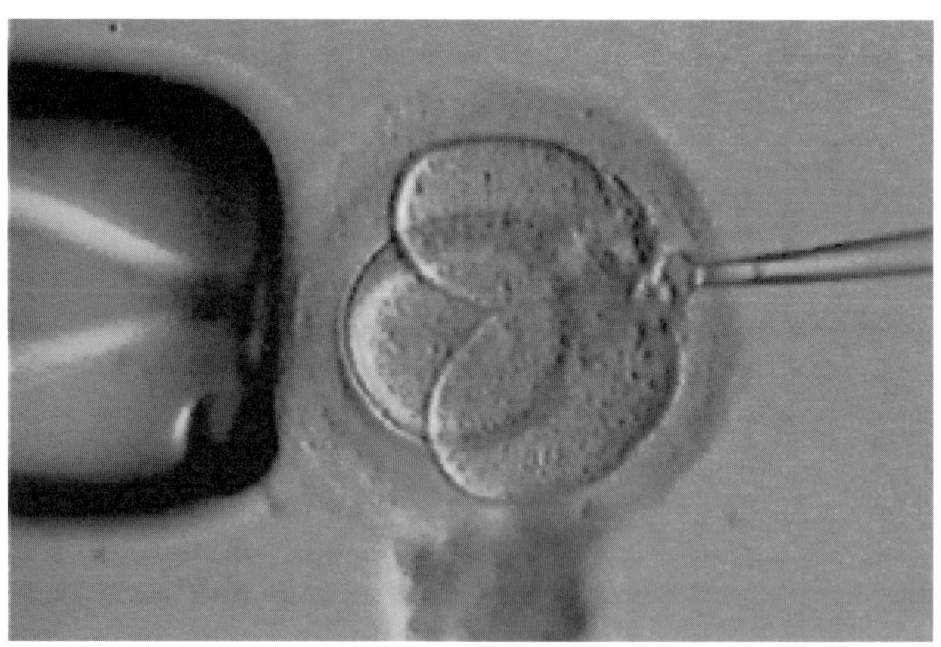

Figure 12.15 In assisted hatching, acid Tyrode's solution is forced under pressure through a blunt micropipette, dissolving a portion of the zona pellucida with a circular motion.

4. The inside of the zona is more difficult to pierce, and the expulsion pressure may need to be increased. The optical system should be optimized for this part of the procedure, as the stream of acid may be relatively invisible, and the piercing of the inside of the zona may be almost imperceptible.
5. Expulsion of the acidic medium should be ceased immediately when the inside of the zona is pierced or softened. Suction is recommended at this point, to aspirate all of the expelled acid solution (the total time to breach the zona should be in the order of 5–7 seconds), and move the embryo to another area of the droplet, away from the acid solution.
6. A small 'inside' hole may be widened mechanically by moving the microneedle through the opening in a tearing motion while continuing gentle suction.
7. Carefully transfer the embryo through the wash droplets, and return to culture for incubation prior to embryo transfer.

Further reading

Bonduelle, M., Legein, J., Buysse, A., Devnaly, P., Van Steirteghem, A.C. & Liebaers, T. (1994) Prospective follow-up study of 55 children born after subzonal insemination and intracytoplasmic sperm injection. *Human Reproduction* **9**: 1765–1769.

Cohen, J. (1992) Zona pellucida micromanipulation and consequences for embryonic development and implantation. In: (J. Cohen, H.F. Malter, B.E. Talansky, J. Grifo, eds), *Micromanipulation of Human Gametes and Embryos*, Raven Press, New York.

DeFelici, M. & Siracusa, G. (1982) 'Spontaneous' hardening of the zona pellucida of mouse oocytes during in vitro culture. *Gamete Research* **6**: 107–112.

Downs, S.M., Schroeder, A.C. & Eppig J.J. (1986) Serum maintains the fertilizability of mouse oocytes matured in vitro by preventing hardening of the zona pellucida. *Gamete Research* **15**: 115–122.

Hamberger, L., Sjögren, A. & Lundin, K. (1995) Microfertilization techniques: choice of correct indications. In: *Fertility and Sterility: A Current Overview* (B. Hedon, J. Bringer, P. Mares, eds), IFFS-95, The Parthenon Publishing Groups, New York, London, pp. 405–408.

Longo F.J. (1981) Changes in the zonae pellucidae and plasmalemmae of aging mouse eggs. *Biological Reproduction* **25**: 299–411.

Nagy, Z.P., Janssenswillen, C., Silber, S., Devroey, P. & Van Steirteghem, A.C. (1995) Using ejaculated, fresh, and frozen-thawed epididymal and testicular spermatozoa gives rise to comparable results after intracytoplasmic injection. *Human Reproduction* **9**: 1743–1748.

Nagy, Z.P., Liu, J., Joris, H., Devroey, P. & Van Steirteghem, A. (1993) Intracytoplasmic single sperm injection of 1-day old unfertilized human oocytes. *Human Reproduction* **8**: 2180–2184.

Nagy, Z.P., Liu, J., Joris, H., Devroey, P., & Van Steirteghem, A.(1993) Time-course of oocyte activation, pronucleus formation and cleavage in human oocytes fertilized by intracytoplasmic sperm injection. *Human Reproduction* **9**: 1743–1748.

Oates, R.D., Cobl, S.M., Harns D.H., Pang, S., Burgess, C.M. & Carson, R.S. (1996) Efficiency of ICSI using intentionally cryopreserved epidymal sperm. *Human Reproduction* **11**: 133–138.

Palermo, G., Joris,.H., Derde, M-P, Camus, M., Devroey, P. & Van Steirteghem, A.C. (1993) Sperm characteristics and outcome of human assisted fertilization by subzonal insemination and intracytoplasmic sperm injection. *Fertility and Sterility* **59:** 826–835.

Palermo, G., Joris,.H., Devroey, P. & Van Steirteghem, A.C. (1992) Pregnancies after intracytoplasmic injection of single spermatozoon into an oocyte. *Lancet* **340:** 17–18.

Silber, S.J., Van Steirteghem, A.C., Liu, J., Nagy, Z., Tournaye, H. & Devroey, P. (1995) High fertilization and pregnancy rate after intracytoplasmic sperm injection with spermatozoa obtained from testicle biopsy. *Human Reproduction* **10:** 148–152.

Van Steirteghem, A.C, Liu, J., Joris, H., Nagy, Z.P., Janssenswillen, C., Tournaye, H., Derde, M-P., Van Assche, E. & Devroey, P. (1993) Higher success rate by intracytoplasmic sperm injection than by subzonal insemination. Report of a second series of 300 consecutive treatment cycles. *Human Reproduction* **8:** 1055–1060.

Van Steirteghem, A., Liu, J., Nagy, P., Joris, H., Staessen, C., Smitz, J., Tournaye, H., Camus, M., Liebaers, I. & Devroey, P. (1995) Microinsemination. In: *Fertility and Sterility: A Current Overview* (B. Hedon, J. Bringer, P. Mares, eds), IFFS-95, The Parthenon Publishing Groups, New York, London, pp. 295–404.

Index

A23187 ionophore 27
acid Tyrode's solution 176, 177
acrosome 19–21, 22, 40–1
   reaction 20, 21, 22, 27, 41
albumin, human serum 81
Alsevers solution 89
amphibia
   embryo micromanipulation 64
   embryogenesis 48, 49
   oocytes 6, 8, 9–10, 11, 13–14
   sperm 5
   sperm–oocyte interaction 22, 25, 34
ampoules, cryopreservation 137, 145
animal pole 8, 11
animal–vegetal (A–V) axis 11–12, 46–7, 49–50
Antheraea 10
antisperm antibodies 86, 88–9
   ICSI 151
   sperm preparation 93
ARIC test 28
artificial insemination (AI)
   farm animals 1, 58–9
   humans 59, 146
Ascaris 38, 50
ascidians
   embryogenesis 48–9
   oocytes 6, 12, 21, 23
   sperm–oocyte interaction 19, 21, 22, 29, 30, 34
assisted hatching (AH) 69, 153, 176–9
asthenozoospermia 96–7, 151
axoneme disorders 151
azoospermia, obstructive 97, 151

'bindin' 20
biopsy, embryo 69, 70, 71, 120–1
birds 6, 8, 48
blastocoel 47, 51
blastocysts 51, 53
   cryopreservation 139–41
blastomeres 46, 47
   assessment of appearance 116, 117
   biopsy 70, 71, 120–1

formation of cell lines 48–50
fragmentation 116, 117, 118–20
microsurgical removal 62
vegetal 49–50
blastula 47
buoyant density
   discontinuous gradient centrifugation 90, 92–4, 95
     mini-gradient method 92, 94
     two-step method 93–4
   isotonic, preparation 93
buserelin (Suprefact) 102, 103, 142

calcium (Ca^{2+})
   in acrosome reaction 27–8
   in oocyte activation 2, 14, 30, 31, 34, 43
Campanularia 25, 26
capacitation 27–8, 40
   in vitro 61
capillary tubing, ICSI microtools 168
carbon dioxide (CO_2) incubators 75, 82
Cdc2 kinase 14
cell lineage formation 48–50
centrifugation
   high-speed, sperm preparation 95
   buoyant density discontinuous gradient 90, 92–4, 95
centrosome 44
chemotaxis, sperm 25–6
chimeras 62, 63
chorion 6, 34
chorionic gonadotrophin, human (hCG) 103, 105, 125
chromosomes
   lampbrush 10
   mixing of female/male 38–9
cleaning routine, IVF laboratory 76
cleavage 46
   assessment after ICSI 159
   holoblastic (complete) 48
   meroblastic (incomplete) 48
   patterns 46–8
   spiral 47

cloning 62, 64–6
co-culture systems, embryo 126–8
coelenterates 3, 6, 13
coitus (mating) 23–4, 39–40
consent 105
cortical reaction, oocyte 31–5, 43
cryopreservation 132–49
  embryos 132–9, 159
    freezing programme 137–8
    materials 135–6
    method 136–9
    selection for 115, 121, 134–5
    thawing 138–9
  oocytes 144
  semen 1, 59, 144–7
    insemination methods 146
    Kryo-10 freezing programme 145–6
    manual 145
    sample preparation 145
    solutions 146–7
cryoprotectants (CPM)
  embryo 133
  semen 59, 145, 146–7
cryptozoospermia 95, 150–1
culture
  co-culture systems 126–8
  equipment required 82–3
  media, *see* media
  quality control tests 78
  systems 80–1, 105–6
cumulus oophorus 6
  cells, in vitro oocyte maturation 60–1
  removal techniques 61, 111–12, 153–4
  retrieved oocytes 107, 108–9
  sperm interaction 27, 40–1
cycle
  monitoring 104
  natural, frozen embryo transfer 142
  treatment 83, 102–5
    frozen embryo transfer 142–3
cyclin 14
Cyclogest 103, 123, 142–3
cytostatic factor (CSF) 31

2-deoxyadenosine 96
density gradients 90, 92–4, 95
desmosomes 50
development, first stages 46–52
diacylglycerol 31–2
dimethyl sulphoxide (DMSO) 134
Discoglossus 22, 26
DNA
  oocyte 10–11
  sperm 44
Drosophila 10, 24

Earle's balanced salt solution (EBSS) 79, 153–4
echinoderms 6, 23, 33
ejaculation 38–40
  disorders 151
  retrograde 98–9, 151
electroejaculation 98–9, 151

electrofusion 65
embryonic stem (ES) cells 63
embryos
  biopsy 69, 70, 71, 120–1
  classification 115–17
  co-culture systems 126–8
  cryopreservation, *see* cryopreservation, embryos
  culture 61, 79
  culture media 78
  dissection 111–12
  early 46–52
    cleavage patterns 46–8
    clinical research 71
    cytoplasmic segregation/cell lineages 48–50
    in mammals 50–2, 53
    micromanipulation 62–6
    nuclear transplantation 62, 64–6
    somatic/germ cell line segregation 50
  frozen-thawed 132–3
    assessment 117–18
    transfer (FET) 141–3
  hatching 52, 54
    assisted (AH) 69, 153, 176–9
  implantation 52, 54
  mosaic 49
  multipronucleate, culture 79
  quality/selection 115–20
  surplus 79, 115, 121, 159
  transfer 120–2
    after ICSI 159
    contraindications 123
    frozen-thawed embryos 141–3
    luteal phase support 123
    procedure 121–2
    selection for 115–20
  see also zygotes
endocrinology
  baseline assessment 102, 104
  reproductive 55–6, 57
epididymis
  sperm aspiration 97, 151
  sperm maturation 16–17
equipment
  ICSI 152–3, 160–1
  IVF laboratory 74–7, 82–3
  microtool preparation 161, 168–70
  sperm preparation 99
  washing procedures 77
erection, penile 39

farm animals 58–66
  artificial insemination 1, 58–9
  in vitro technologies 60–6, 70–1
feeder cells 126–7
fertilization 2–3, 19–44
  cone 37
  failure, after ICSI 159–60
  membrane 33–5
  potential 27–31, 43
  see also sperm–oocyte interaction
fish
  embryos 48

Index

oocytes 5–6, 8
   sperm–oocyte interaction 21, 23, 25, 26, 35
flow cytometry sorters 70
fluorescent in situ hybridization (FISH) 70, 113
follicle cells 9
follicle stimulating hormone (FSH) 13, 55, 56, 57
   ovarian stimulation 102, 103, 104
follicles, ovarian 14–15
   antral (Graafian) 14
   flushing media 78
   pre-antral 14
   primordial 14
   recruitment 14
four-well plates 106, 111
fragmentation, blastomere 115–17, 118–20
FSH, see follicle stimulating hormone
fucose 19, 20

gamete intra-fallopian transfer (GIFT) 122–4
   procedure 124
   sperm preparation 89–96
gametes
   heterogeneity 2–3
   see also oocytes; sperm(atozoa)
gametogenesis 3, 5
gap junctions 9, 14, 50
gene transfer methods 62–3
genetic diagnosis, pre-implantation 69, 70, 71, 120–1
germ cells, segregation from somatic cells 50
germinal vesicle 8, 12
   breakdown 13
   in retrieved oocytes 106–8
Gestone 103, 123, 142–3
GIFT, see gamete intra-fallopian transfer
globozoospermia 98, 151
glycerol 134, 139–40, 147
glycoproteins
   sperm 16–17, 42–3
   vitelline coat 19, 21–2
   zona pellucida 42–3
GnRH, see gonadotrophin releasing hormone
gonadotrophin releasing hormone (GnRH; LHRH) 55–6, 57
   analogues 59, 102–5, 142
gonadotrophins 55, 56
   ovarian stimulation 102, 103, 104
   ovulation induction 59
Gonal F 102, 103
granulosa cells 14, 15
   in vitro oocyte maturation 60–1
   retrieved oocytes 106
growth hormone genes 63

heparin 61, 79
HEPES-buffered human tubal fluid (HTF) medium 177
HEPES-containing media 79, 106, 154
hormone replacement therapy (HRT) 143
hormones
   controlling reproduction 55–6, 57
   in oocyte maturation 13

human chorionic gonadotrophin (hCG) 103, 104, 125
humidity 75
hyaluronidase (hyalase) 40, 109, 153–4, 155
hypothalamus 55, 57

ICSI, see intracytoplasmic sperm injection
IMMAC power cleaner 168
immunological factors 151
in vitro fertilization (IVF)
   farm animals 60–1
   laboratory 73–83
   procedure 110–11
   scoring on day 1: 111–15
      embryo dissection 111–12
      re-insemination 114–15
      technique 113–14
   semen cryopreservation 144
   sperm preparation 89–96
   transport 124–6
incubators 75, 82–3
infection control 105–6
infertility
   idiopathic 152
   male factor 85, 150–1
inhibins 56, 57
injection dish, ICSI 154–5, 156
inner cell mass 51, 54
insects
   embryos 48
   oocytes 8, 10, 35
   sperm 5, 24
insemination
   artificial, see artificial insemination
   frozen-thawed sperm 146
   intrauterine, see intrauterine insemination
   microsurgical techniques 67–71
   oocyte, in vitro 110–11
intracytoplasmic sperm injection (ICSI) 67–9, 85, 150–60
   adjustment of Narishige manipulators 161–7
   assessment of fertilization/cleavage 159
   facilities and equipment 152–3, 160–1
   indications 150–2
   injection procedure 157–8
   microtool preparation 167–76
   no fertilization after 159–60
   oocyte preparation/handling 153–4
   preparation for injection 154–6
   sperm preparation 94, 95, 97–8
   sperm selection/immobilization 156–7
   transport 160
intrauterine insemination
   frozen-thawed sperm 144, 146
   sperm preparation 89–96
ions
   in acrosome reaction 28–9
   in oocyte activation 2–3, 27–31
IVF, see in vitro fertilization

jelly layer, oocyte 21, 26, 35
junctions, intercellular 9, 14, 50

Kartagener's syndrome   151
Kruger criteria   87
Kryo 10, *see* Planer Kryo 10
KSB buffer   146, 147

laboratory, in vitro fertilization   73–83
    culture media   78, 83
    daily cleaning routine   76
    equipment and facilities   74–6, 82–3
    quality control procedures   79
    tissue culture systems   80–2
    washing procedures   77
lampbrush chromosomes   10
latent period   34
layering method, sperm preparation   90–1, 95
LH, *see* luteinizing hormone
lipid peroxidation   90, 92
luteal phase support   103, 123, 142–3
luteinizing hormone (LH)   13, 55, 56, 57
    baseline assessment   103
    oocyte maturation and   109–10
    surge   15, 59
luteinizing hormone releasing hormone (LHRH),
    see gonadotrophin releasing hormone

MacLeod scale   87
macromeres   47
male factor infertility   85, 150–1
mammals
    embryo micromanipulation   62–6
    embryogenesis   50–2, 53
    implantation   52, 54
    mating   23–4
    oocytes   5–6, 8, 10, 13–14
    oogenesis   14–15
    reproductive endocrinology   55–6, 57
    sperm–oocyte interaction   19, 21, 25, 29, 36–8, 38–44
    spermatogenesis   15–17
marine invertebrates
    oocytes   5, 13
    spawning   23
    sperm   26
    sperm–oocyte interaction   38–44
maternal serum   81
mating   23–4, 38
maturation promoting factor (MPF)   14, 31
media
    assisted hatching   177
    commercial suppliers   83
    culture, *see* culture media
    embryo cryopreservation   135–6
    embryo culture   78
    follicular flushing   78
    ICSI   153–4
    oocyte maturation   60–1
    oocyte retrieval   106
    semen cryopreservation   146–7
    serum supplements   80–1
    sperm preparation   86, 90–1
meiosis   3, 4
    in oogenesis   3–5, 6, 12–13, 15
    in spermatogenesis   3, 16
menstrual cycle, *see* cycle
mesomeres   47
messenger RNA (mRNA)   10
metabolic activity, oocyte maturation   13–14
1-methyl-adenine   13
Metrodin HP   102, 103
microbeveller   169
microforge   169, 175–6
microgrinder   169
micromanipulation
    farm animals   61–6
    human clinical use   67–71, 109
    techniques   150–79
micromanipulators
    adjustment   161–7
    use   155–6
micromeres   47
micropipette puller (MPP11)   169
micropyle   22–3
microsurgical epididymal sperm aspiration (MESA)   97, 151
microtools   152–3, 155–6
    equipment for making   161, 168–70
    preparation   167–76
    technique of use   157–8
    see also pipettes
microvilli, oocyte   9, 36–7
mixed antiglobulin reaction (MAR) test   88–9
molluscs   6, 12, 47
morula   51, 53
Mos protein kinase   14
mosaic embryos   49

nafarelin (Synarel)   102, 103, 142
Narishige manipulators, adjustment   161–7
needle dissection, inseminated oocytes   111
nematodes   24, 50
Nereis   6, 34
Nikon/Narishige manipulators, adjustment   161–7
nuclear transplantation, early embryos   62, 64–6
nurse cells   10

oestradiol   56, 57
    baseline assessment   102, 103
    in stimulated cycle   105
    treatment   142, 143
oestrous cycle   59
oil   82
    equilibriated   80
    microdroplets under   106, 110–11
oligospermia, extreme   97, 150
oncology   151
oocyte/cumulus complex (OCC) assessment   106–10
oocytes
    activation   2, 27–31, 43
    atretic   108, 109
    cell cycle regulation   27–31
    cortex   12
    cortical reaction   31–5, 43
    cortical reorganization   35–6

Index

cryopreservation   144
culture   79, 106
cumulus-corona removal   61, 112, 153–4
fertilizable life   26
follicle cells   9
growth   8–9
ICSI, *see* intracytoplasmic sperm injection
immature   106–8
in vitro insemination   110–11
informational molecules   9–11
luteinized   108, 109
maturation   3–5, 12–14, 109–10
   assessment of status   107–9, 154, 155
   in vitro   1, 60–1
meiosis   3–5, 6, 12–13, 15
micromanipulation, *see* micromanipulation
morphology   5–6
nuclear transplantation   62, 64–6
post-mature   108–9
pre-ovulatory   107–8
quality assessment   107–9, 154
regional organization   11–12
retrieval (OCR)   107–10
   farm animals   60
   human clinical protocol   103–4
sperm interaction, *see* sperm–oocyte interaction
see also zygotes
oogenesis   3, 5, 8–15
   in mammals   14–15
ovarian stimulation
   monitoring   105
   schedule   102, 103, 104
ovaries
   endocrine control   56, 57
   ultrasound assessment   103
ovens, heat sterilization   169
ovulation   15
   induction   59, 103, 105
oxygen species, reactive   90, 92

paraffin, semen layering under   95
paraplegia   151
partial zona dissection (PZD)   67, 68, 69, 153, 176–9
PCP7 Plug board   168
pellet and swim-up method, sperm preparation   91–2
pentoxifylline   96
perivitelline space   34, 35, 36
   fragments in   118
   sperm injection (SUZI)   67, 68, 69
peroxidative damage, sperm   90, 92
pH
   acrosome reaction and   27
   in oocyte activation   29–30
   sperm preparations   90
phenol red   136
phosphate buffered saline (PBS)   135
pigments, oocyte   11
pipettes   77
   ICSI holding   152–3, 157, 168
      equipment for making   168–70

      manipulation   155–6
      pulling   170–1, 172
   ICSI injection   152–3, 157–8, 168
      equipment for making   168–70
      manipulation   155–6
      pulling   173–4
   narrow gauge
      cumulus removal   112, 154
      preparation   112–13
   pullers   169
   pulling techniques   170–5
   storage containers   169
   washing procedure   77
pituitary hormones   13, 55, 56, 57
Planer Kryo 10
   embryo freezing programmes   137–8, 140
   operation   140–1
   semen freezing programme   145–6
plasma membrane
   fusion of oocyte/sperm   36–7, 42–3
   oocyte   22–3, 36
plasms   48–9
plastics, tissue culture   82
platelets   8
polar bodies
   after ICSI   159
   oocyte maturity and   107
polycystic ovaries (PCO)   102
polymerase chain reaction (PCR)   70
polyspermy   24
   blocks   36, 43–4
polyvinylpyrrolidone (PVP)   94, 97, 153, 154
potassium (K^+)
   acrosome reaction and   27
   in oocyte activation   2, 27
   sperm motility and   26
pre-embryo   51
pre-ovulatory phase   15
pregnancy rates   143
   embryo co-cultures   127
   frozen embryo transfer   132, 143
   GIFT   122–3
progesterone   56
   baseline assessment   102, 104
   luteal phase support   103, 123, 142–3
pronuclei
   formation   37–8, 44
   fusion   37–8
   injection techniques   62–3
   scoring   113–14, 159
1,2-propanediol (PROH)   133, 134, 135, 137
protamines   44

quality control (QC)   78–9

re-insemination   114–15
red blood cells (RBCs), preparation   89
regulation   49
reptiles   6, 8, 48
ribonucleic acids (RNAs), oocyte   9–10
ribosomes/ribosomal RNA   9–10
'rolling', inseminated oocytes   112

sea urchins
  embryogenesis 46–7, 49
  oocytes 11–12, 19
    activation 27, 31–2, 33–4, 35
    meiosis 3, 6, 13
    microinsemination 67
    sperm 5
    sperm–oocyte interaction 21, 24, 25, 36, 37
second messengers 2, 41
sedimentation method, sperm preparation 95
semen
  analysis 85–9
  collection 58, 85–6
  cryopreservation 1, 59, 144–7
  ejaculation 39–40
  excessive debris 98
  liquefaction 86
  volume 58, 86
  see also sperm(atozoa)
seminal plasma 90
serum
  maternal 81
  supplements 80–1
sex determination 69–70
shells 6
somatic cells, segregation from germ cells 50
spawning 23
sperm(atozoa)
  100% abnormal heads 98
  activation 2, 24–9
  capacitation, see capacitation
  chemotaxis 25
  density 86–7
  duration of fertility 27
  epididymal aspiration 97, 151
  epididymal maturation 16–17
  high-speed centrifugation/washing 95
  ICSI, see intracytoplasmic sperm injection
  morphology 5, 40, 87–8
  motility 24–5, 86–7
    chemical enhancement 96
    no motile 98
  nucleus decondensation 44
  numbers 23–4, 58–9
  pellet and swim-up 91–2
  preparation 89–99
    equipment/materials 99
    ICSI 94, 97–9
    IVF/GIFT/intrauterine insemination 89–96
    methods 99
    retrograde ejaculation/electroejaculation 98–9
  progression 87
  sedimentation/layering under paraffin 95
  separating X and Y 69–70
  sticky 98
  survival test 79
  swim-up/layering 90–1, 95
  testicular extraction 97, 151
  transport in female tract 39
  see also insemination; semen

sperm–oocyte interaction 2, 19–44
  factors limiting 21–4
  formation/fusion of pronuclei 37–8
  major events 19
  in mammals 19, 21, 26, 27, 36–44
  oocyte activation 29–32
  oocyte cortical reaction/reorganization 31–6
  prior sperm activation 24–9
  zygote nucleus formation 36–8
sperm:oocyte ratios 23–4, 36, 40, 41
spermatogenesis 3, 5
  in mammals 15–17
starfish 13–14, 19, 21
straws, cryopreservation 136, 137, 145
subzonal sperm injection (SUZI) 67, 68, 69
sucrose 133, 135
superovulation 59, 102–6
  preparation for each case 105–6
  protocol 102–4
  in transport IVF 125
supplies
  IVF laboratory 76
  sperm preparation 99
Suprefact (buserelin) 102, 103, 142
swim-up methods, sperm preparation 90–2
symmetry, bilateral 12
Synarel (nafarelin) 102, 103, 142

temperature
  oocyte/embryo culture 80
  in vitro fertilization and 61
teratozoospermia 151
testis
  endocrine control 56, 57
  sperm aspiration (TESA) 97, 151
testosterone 56
transgenic animals 62–3
transport ICSI 160
transport IVF 124–6
trophectoderm cells 51, 54
trypsinization 128
twins, monozygotic 52
Tyrode's solution, acid 176, 177

ultrasound
  assessment 103, 104
  oocyte retrieval 103–4
uterus
  implantation of embryo 52, 54
  ultrasound assessment 103
Utrogestan 105, 123, 143

vagina, artificial 58
vas deferens
  congenital absence 151
  post-inflammatory obstruction 151
vegetal pole 8, 11
Vero cell lines 127
vitelline block 43
vitelline coat 6, 9, 19–21
  elevation 34–5
  sperm binding 19–20

Index

washing procedures, IVF laboratory   77
water, purified   77, 83
World Health Organization (WHO)   85

Xenopus   9–10, 22

yolk   8–9, 48, 147

zona pellucida   6, 14, 15
   assisted hatching (AH)   69, 153, 176–9
   damage, in cumulus removal   112
   early embryo   51–2
   partial drilling (PZD)   67, 68, 69, 153, 176–9
   sperm interaction   41, 42

zona radiata   9
zona reaction   35, 43
ZP1   42
ZP2   42
ZP3   40, 42
zygotes   50–1
   cleavage   46–8
   cryopreservation   134–5
   ICSI   159
   micromanipulation   62–6
   nucleus formation   36–7
   pronucleus scoring   113–14
   see also embryos; oocytes